YOUR PERSONAL INFORMATION CHANNEL

Here is the one and only TV book that offers an irresistible show of knowledge on every page. Here is more than you ever dreamed about the lives of the stars and the stories of the shows on the home screen and off.

Here are the performers as familiar as old friends. Here are the programs you can now view with greater insight and pleasure than ever before. This is the book of lists that everyone will put at the *top* of the list, for nonstop reading and endless browsing delight.

THE SIGNET BOOK OF TV LISTS

THE SIGNET BOOK OF TV LISTS

by Jeff Rovin

A SIGNET BOOK
NEW AMERICAN LIBRARY
TIMES MIRROR

NAL BOOKS ARE AVAILABLE AT QUANTITY DISCOUNTS WHEN USED TO PROMOTE PRODUCTS OR SERVICES. FOR INFORMATION PLEASE WRITE TO PREMIUM MARKETING DIVISION, THE NEW AMERICAN LIBRARY, INC., 1633 BROADWAY, NEW YORK, NEW YORK 10019.

SIGNET TRADEMARK REG. U.S. PAT. OFF. AND FOREIGN COUNTRIES
REGISTERED TRADEMARK—MARCA REGISTRADA
HECHO EN CHICAGO, U.S.A.

SIGNET, SIGNET CLASSICS, MENTOR, PLUME, MERIDIAN AND NAL BOOKS are published by The New American Library, Inc., 1633 Broadway, New York, New York 10019

First Printing, August, 1982

1 2 3 4 5 6 7 8 9

PRINTED IN THE UNITED STATES OF AMERICA

Dedications usually mean nothing to a reader, nothing in fact to *anyone,* save the author and her/his spouse, mother-who-believed, dog, literary hero, fourth-grade teacher, or mentor. In this case, however, the author is taking the liberty of dedicating a book to some people who are no longer with us, but who have done a great deal to contribute to our years of TV enjoyment. They are missed, and can be neither replaced nor underrated.

Ross Martin
Paddy Chayefsky
Bob Crane
Carl Betz
Richard Long
Milburn Stone
Al Hodge
Barbara Colby
Rod Serling
Gracie Allen

Leo G. Carroll
Jack Soo
Will Geer
Diana Hyland
David Janssen
Larry Blyden
George Reeves
William Boyd
Dan Blocker

PREFACE

A word about the dates and format of this book.

The dates which follow each program are the *seasons* of the show's original run. Some programs, like *Hawk,* returned years later when its star became popular or a summer fill-in was needed. These reruns have not been included.

The seasons are, further, *not* the same as the *years* the show was seen on the air. *Twelve O'Clock High* aired from 1964–1967. However, its final season was 1966/67. In the shorthand we have used, that's printed simply as 1966. In most cases, however, original episodes in a series were aired into the following year.

For the purposes of this book, once a program's dates have been cited, we don't repeat them. We'd have a considerable clutter if we did, thus defeating the whole purpose of a sleek and streamlined, easy-to-scan book of lists!

INTRODUCTION

To list all the list books which have appeared over the past few years would take—well, it would take quite a list in itself. This makes the third one Signet has published. The first two were about motion pictures; now we're tackling television.

Actually, TV cries out for lists. For one thing, there has been so much programming on TV throughout its thirty-four-year commercial history that lists are virtually the *only* way to keep track of what's been on, who played who, and similar data. Too, TV is a fun, diverting, informative, sometimes trivial, always resilient medium: this book is, we feel, an accurate translation of those qualities to book form.

Anyone with access to a complete run of *TV Guide* magazines can concoct a book of TV lists. We think this book is more than that. There are firsthand memories here: lines from the theme songs of TV shows long since vanished into the ether; cultural footnotes observed by a product of the TV generation; in short, not the sort of material you'll find in other television books —not even in the *TV Guide* crossword puzzle.

Most of the lists compiled for this book draw from prime-time network series. Syndicated programs are worthy of an entire book in themselves, and daytime shows *several* volumes. The few exceptions, like *The Adventures of Superman,* are cited only because their impact rivaled that of the network shows. This book is, finally, intended as something of a romp through TV history. Rather than put together an encyclopedia, we've compiled a "memory-jogger," a casual collection of TV trivia. Hope you enjoy it!

JEFF ROVIN

Tempest in a Teapot

Major motion-picture stars who have done made-for-TV movies:

Elizabeth Taylor in *Divorce Hers* (1973), being one view of a decaying marriage.

Richard Burton in *Divorce His* (1973), a companion film to the above.

Bette Davis in *Madame Sin* (1972), the first of several home-screen efforts for the star.

Joan Crawford in *Night Gallery* (1969), in one of three stories in this anthology film. The sequence was directed by Steven Spielberg, age nineteen, who went on to direct *Jaws* in 1975. *Night Gallery* was successful enough to inspire a popular series of the same name.

Cliff Robertson in *My Father's House* (1975), about the victim of a heart attack. Robertson also played astronaut Buzz Aldrin in *Return to Earth* the following year, based on the hero's breakdown after the Apollo XI moon landing.

Gloria Swanson enjoyed a strange rapport with insects in *The Killer Bees* (1974), in the best film of this type, TV or theatrical.

Helen Hayes in *Do Not Fold, Spindle, or Mutilate* (1971), a bit of fluff about nasty, prank-pulling old ladies. Myrna Loy was also in on the silliness.

Ray Milland and Gene Tierny both in *Daughter of the Mind* (1969), about a man led to believe that his daughter is trying to communicate with him from beyond the grave.

Natalie Wood in *The Cracker Factory* (1979), based on the best-seller about a housewife who has a breakdown.

Kim Novak in *Satan's Triangle* (1975), a Bermuda Triangle fantasy-horror story.

Susan Hayward in *Say Goodbye, Maggie Cole* (1972), the story of a compassionate physician who works in the slums.

Autobiographies written by TV personalities:

The Confessions of Phoebe Tyler by Ruth Warrick
I Am Not Spock by Leonard Nimoy
This I Believe by Lawrence Welk
My Own Story by Phil Donahue
Merv by Merv Griffin
My Story by Mike Douglas
I Ain't Down Yet by Gale Storm
The Camera Never Blinks by Dan Rather

TV series inspired by successful motion pictures:

Planet of the Apes (1974), more adventures among the monkeys
Breaking Away (1980), small-town teen antics
Adam's Rib (1973), about married attorneys
Logan's Run (1977), teens on the run from totalitarians in the future
Bob & Carol & Ted & Alice (1973), toned down the sexual escapades of the feature-film couples
Foul Play (1980), a young couple solving crimes
Paper Moon (1974), about a con man and his preteen daughter
Peyton Place (1964–1968), the soap-opera doings in a small New England town
Going My Way (1962–1963), about an iconoclastic young clergy member
Voyage to the Bottom of the Sea (1964–1967), the further adventures of the nuclear submarine *Seaview*
The Wackiest Ship in the Army (1965), did not fare as well as the *Seaview*, in this comedy set on the high seas of World War II.
Mr. Lucky (1959), the adventures of a gambling ship operator
Mr. Smith Goes to Washington (1962), the gosh-shucks Fess Parker replacing Jimmy Stewart
Operation Petticoat (1977), nurses and sailors on a World War II submarine
Alice (1976–present), based on the film *Alice Doesn't Live Here Any More*, which won star Ellen Burstyn an Academy Award as a waitress and single mother
Serpico (1976), both film and TV show deriving from

a book written by a former NY policeman about his experiences

Shaft (1973), with Richard Roundtree repeating as a private eye

*M*A*S*H* (1972–present), doings at an army hospital in Korea, primarily comedic

Anna and the King (1972), which was *The King and I* without the music

The Courtship of Eddie's Father (1969–1971), with Bill Bixby instead of Glenn Ford as the widower with a son

Shane (1966), the return of the taciturn cowpoke

National Velvet (1960–1961), yet more horsin' around

Room for One More (1962), a couple which keeps on adopting kids in need

Hondo (1967), a soldier in prestatehood Arizona

Father of the Bride (1961), a sit com remotely related to the Spencer Tracy film

No Time for Sergeants (1964), being an air-force comedy

Love Story (1973), stories of the same sort as the tearful film

The Greatest Show on Earth (1963), adventures beneath the big top

The Ghost and Mrs. Muir (1968–1969), a sea captain haunting a widow

Gidget (1965), based on the successful series of films about a precocious teen

Dr. Kildare (1961–1965), from the series about a young medic

Topper (1953–1955), continuing the adventures of the ghostly Kerbys and their living associate Cosmo Topper; inspired by a trio of films and, earlier, a series of novels

Naked City (1958–1962), covering the 7,999,999 stories not touched upon in the motion picture

House Calls (1980–present), continuing with Wayne

Rogers and Lynn Redgrave what Walter Matthau and Glenda Jackson had begun

The Paper Chase (1978), being the conflict between Professor Kingsfield and James T. Hart

Twelve O'Clock High (1964–1966), at war with the air force and Brigadier General Savage

The Bad News Bears (1979), more adventures of the misfit little-league team

Movie stars who had elected to star in weekly TV series—usually with disastrous results:

Yul Brynner starred in *Anna and the King*, a situation comedy based on his blockbuster Oscar-winner *The King and I* (1956). The 1972 series lasted two months.

Henry Fonda did *The Smith Family*, playing Detective Sergeant Chad Smith, a look at the lawman's home life. The series ran from January 1971 to June 1972.

Jimmy Stewart used his folksy screen persona to play lawyer Billy Jim Hawkins in *Hawkins*, but the translation didn't work. The show lasted under a year, dying in the fall of 1974.

Doris Day had one of the most successful such shows of them all, *The Doris Day Show*, running from September 1968 until September 1973. She played widow Doris Martin.

Anthony Quinn endured a short, painful death on TV as Mayor Thomas Jefferson Alcala in *The Man and the City*, which expired in January of 1972, less than three months after it went on the air.

Mickey Rooney gave *Mickey* his best, playing an Omaha-based coast-guard officer, but the program survived only from September 1964 to January of the following year.

Rock Hudson was luckier than most of his peers, scoring heavily with *McMillan and Wife*, a police-show-cum-soap-opera which ran from 1971–1976.

Ernest Borgnine got good ratings but did little for his thus-far-distinguished career by playing Lt. Cdr. Quinton McHale in *McHale's Navy* for four years, beginning in 1962.

Robert Taylor fared moderately trying to bring his rugged charisma to the home tube in *The Detectives* (1959–1961). For its last season, the series was renamed *Robert Taylor's Detectives* in an attempt to capitalize on the star's name.

Gene Kelly, perhaps the cinema's greatest dancer, took a pratfall as Father O'Malley in *Going My Way* (1962).

Tony Curtis, despite the publicity of a pot bust, failed to catch the public fancy in *The Persuaders.*

Barbara Stanwyck did not do much better than ex-husband Robert Taylor with her one-season *The Barbara Stanwyck Show* (1960), but improved in *The Big Valley* (1965–1968).

Ray Milland came to the home screen in *Meet Mr. McNutley* (1953–1954), which was retitled *The Ray Milland Show* and still went off the air.

Shirley MacLaine went on location around the globe as a reporter in *Shirley's World* (1971–1972), but audiences weren't up for the trip.

Julie Andrews brought song and dance of a high caliber to TV in *The Julie Andrews Hour,* but audiences preferred her as Maria von Trapp. She came to TV in 1972, and was gone by 1973.

Boris Karloff managed to come up with one of the few enduring shows, hosting and frequently starring in the anthology series *Thriller* (1960–1961) which, though comparatively short-lived, enjoys wide popularity in syndication.

David Niven, who'd done a short-lived anthology series in the fifties, returned in the expensive *The Rogues* (1964), failing in the good company of fellow film greats Charles Boyer and Gig Young.

Shirley Temple, like Boris Karloff, found a successful medium of transition from film to TV hosting the anthology series *Shirley Temple's Storybook* (1959–1960) in which she sometimes appeared.

Judy Garland, one of the most revered talents of the century, could nonetheless not quite cut it on TV and her much-ballyhooed weekly variety series, *The Judy Garland Show*, was gone one year after its 1963 debut, yet another casualty of the steamroller known as *Bonanza.* It was not until the coming of *The Smothers Brothers Comedy Hour* that that durable old warhorse was knocked down to size.

TV's great and not-so-great duos:

The Sonny and Cher Comedy Hour (1971–1973)
Pete and Gladys (1960–1961)
Mork and Mindy (1978–present)
Laverne & Shirley (1976–present)
Starsky and Hutch (1975–1978)
Rosetti and Ryan (1977)
Holmes and Yo-Yo (1976)
Donny and Marie (1976–1978)
Mr. T and Tina (1976)
Rowan and Martin's Laugh-In (1968–1972)
Alias Smith and Jones (1971–1972)
Joe and Valerie (1978)
The Adventures of Ozzie and Harriet (1952–1965)
Marilyn McCoo and Billy Davis Jr. Show (1977)
Roy Rogers and Dale Evans Show (1962)
Fibber McGee and Molly (1959)
The George Burns and Gracie Allen Show (1950–1957)
Ethel and Albert (1953–1955)
Mary Kay and Johnny (1947–1949)
Shields and Yarnell (1977)
Marge and Jeff (1953)

Cartoon series which have been aired in prime time to attract an adult audience:

The Flintstones (1960–1965), *The Honeymooners* set in the cave days

The Jetsons (1962), a futuristic version of *The Flintstones,* and unsuccessful

The Bullwinkle Show (1961), Rocky and Bullwinkle were never kids stuff, but this prime-time airing of the popular daytime cartoons failed

Jonny Quest (1964), an adventure series with lifelike animation

My World and Welcome to It (1969–1971), James Thurber's stories about middle-class boredom, with cartoonist William Windom coexisting in real life and in his cartoon works

Where's Huddles (1970), a series about animated football players

Top Cat (1961), Arnold Stang was the voice of a streetwise alley cat; though the show did not work for adults, it was proven a resilient kids' show

Matty's Funday Funnies (1959–1961), originally populated by characters from the Harvey line of comics, such as Little Audrey and Casper the Friendly Ghost; later taken over by Beany and Cecil (the Seasick Sea Serpent)

The Famous Adventures of Mr. Magoo (1964), starring the nearsighted character as the protagonist in famous works of literature and legend

The Bugs Bunny Show (1960–1961), the prime-time airing of the theatrically released cartoons. *The Bugs Bunny/Roadrunner Show* came to prime time briefly in 1976

Calvin and the Colonel (1961), a *Pogo*esque series about animals who have migrated from the south to the north and must make adjustments to industrial, urban society; much satire

Shows with a hue in their title:

White Shadow (1978–1980)
The Green Hornet (1966)
Green Acres (1965–1970)
Coronet Blue (1967)
The Blue Knight (1975)
The Red Skelton Show (1951–1970)
The Red Buttons Show (1952–1954)
Black Saddle (1959)
Blue Light (1966)

TV shows with interrogatory names:

Who Do You Trust? (1956–1963), the Johnny Carson game show
Do You Trust Your Wife? (1956), Edgar Bergen's quiz show
It's a Business? (1952), about music publishers in the early 1900s
Who's the Boss (1954), a quiz show featuring the secretaries of famous people
Who's There? (1952), guessing the identity of famous people
What's My Line? (1950–1966), guessing peoples' occupations
Why? (1953), a quiz show where panel is given the who, what, when, and where, and must figure out why.
Who Said That? (1948–1954), identifying quotes
Where Was I? (1952), identifying places through photos
What's the Story (1951–1954), guessing current events through clues
What's Happening (1976–1979), comedic youths growing up in the big city
What's It All About, World? (1969), satirical look at current events
What's It For? (1957), deducing what odd inventions do
Who's Watching the Kids (1978), a lighthearted look at growing up in Vegas
Where's Huddles? (1970), a cartoon about pro footballers
What's Your Bid? (1953), an auction TV show

What Really Happened to the Class of '65? (1977)
What Do You Have in Common (1954), panelists with something in common, only they have to figure out what it is
Car 54, Where Are You? (1961–1962), Toody and Muldoon on patrol

Characters or series which have had more than one incarnation:

Blondie (1957 and 1968): the comic strip came to television twice, with Pamela Britton and Patricia Harty as Blondie, respectively, and Arthur Lake and Will Hutchins as Dagwood.

Buck Rogers (1950 and 1979–1980): the hero of the twenty-fifth century was played by both Kem Dibbs and Robert Pastene; and then by Gil Gerard.

Perry Mason (1957–1965 and 1973): starring Raymond Burr the first time out, and Monte Markham subsequently. Markham, incidentally, gave up a part in the hit Broadway musical *Irene* to do the swiftly canceled series; that, as they say, is show biz.

Ellery Queen (1950–1958 and 1975): a whole crew of people played Queen in the initial run: John Hart, Lee Bowman, George Nader, and Lee Philips; Jim Hutton had the role all to himself in the seventies.

The Saint (1967–1968 and 1980): Roger Moore made a name for himself; Ian Oglivy was unable to do the same.

The Hardy Boys (1955–1958, on-and-off, and 1977–1978): featured on *The Mickey Mouse Club*, starring Tim Considine and Tommy Kirk; Joe and Frank were subsequently portrayed by Shaun Cassidy and Parker Stevenson.

The Price Is Right (1957–1963 and 1972–present): Bill Cullen hosted this game show during its first run; Bob Barker is in charge now.

That was the warning which greeted viewers at the beginning of every episode of *The Outer Limits*, TV's innovative science-fiction series. The show ran for two seasons, 1963–1965, and featured some of the weirdest stories ever aired. Here is a complete listing of the programs:

"The Galaxy Being": Cliff Robertson as a scientist who brings a creature to earth from a distant galaxy using his TV set.
"The One Hundred Days of the Dragon": Asian tyrant, able to mold his features, impersonates an American presidential candidate.
"The Architects of Fear": Robert Culp as an artificially created monster, whose presence is supposed to rally earth around a common foe.
"The Man with the Power": A college professor becomes a telekinetic.
"The Sixth Finger": A man is pushed far ahead on the evolutionary scale and becomes a supermind.
"The Man Who Was Never Born": Martin Landau comes from the future to prevent a holocaust, inadvertently making his own birth impossible and vanishing.
"O.B.I.T.": Aliens create a bug to spy on humans.
"The Human Factor": Two men's minds are switched by accident.
"Corpus Earthling": A pair of rocks plot to take over the earth.
"Nightmare": Earth people captured by aliens during a war become POWs.
"It Crawled Out of the Woodwork": A dustball becomes a monster.

"The Borderland": An adventure in the mirror-image fourth dimension.

"Tourist Attraction": A Loch Ness-type monster discovered in South America.

"The Zanti Misfits": Alien prisoners are exiled on earth.

"The Mice": An alien-exchange program with earth.

"Controlled Experiment": Martians investigate an earth murder.

"Don't Open Till Doomsday": An alien dogs a pair of honeymooners.

"Z-z-z-z-z": A queen bee becomes a human to mate with a scientist.

"The Invisibles": An alien invasion plot investigated by government secret agents.

"The Bellero Shield": A space monster on earth holes up behind an indestructible shield.

"The Children of Spider County": An alien sires superbrilliant earth children.

"Specimen: Unknown": Marauding mushrooms.

"Second Chance": An amusement-park spaceship really blasts off.

"Moonstone": A living globe menaces a moon colony.

"The Mutant": A silver rain turns a sane man into a murdering lunatic.

"The Guests": A house where time stands still.

"Fun and Games": An earth couple battles an alien for the amusement of third-party extraterrestrials.

"The Special One": Earth children are used by an alien in an effort to take over the planet.

"A Feasibility Study": A small section of a city is mysteriously transported to another world.

"Production and Decay of Strange Particles": A faulty nuclear reactor turns loose creatures made of radiation.

"The Chameleon": Robert Duvall as a government agent who infiltrates an alien spaceship.

"The Form of Things Unknown": A machine is invented which can stop time and revive the dead.

"Soldier": A future soldier is brought to the present, his animosity intact.

"Cold Hands, Warm Heart": William Shatner as an astronaut who, returned from Venus, cannot get warm.

"Behold, Eck!": Special glasses reveal the existence of a two-dimensional creature.

"Expanding Human": Drugs which stretch human awareness.

"Demon with a Glass Hand": Humankind is entirely encoded onto a strand of wire placed in the hand of a robot, who must protect his treasure against alien invaders.

"Cry of Silence": Malevolent tumbleweeds.

"The Invisible Enemy": Adam West menaced by a monster on Mars.

"Wolf 359": A planet is created in miniature in a lab, its evolution greatly accelerated, to determine where humanity will end up.

"I, Robot": A robot is placed on trial for murder. Leonard Nimoy co-stars as a reporter.

"The Inheritors": Children are spirited from earth by benevolent aliens.

"Keeper of the Purple Twilight": An alien exchanges his vast intellect for the chance to experience human emotions.

"The Duplicate Man": A rampaging, monstrous Megasoid on-the-loose in suburbia of the twenty-first century.

"Counterweight": A simulated space flight wherein six astronauts are joined by an alien stowaway.

"The Brain of Colonel Barham": A bodyless brain is determined to be the perfect astronaut.

"The Premonition": Time slows down for a couple so that they can somehow engineer a way to save the life of their son, who is about to be run over by a truck.

"The Probe": Plane-crash survivors find themselves in a chamber in the middle of nowhere.

Movies which have been made by stitching together episodes of TV series:

The Venetian Affair (1967): built from segments of *The Man from U.N.C.L.E.*, along with seven other features

Recoil (1963): *The Detectives*, starring Robert Taylor, was used for this film

The Legend of Custer (1968): episodes one and two of the TV show of the same name

Tarzan's Jungle Rebellion (1970) and *Tarzan's Deadly Silence* (1970): both from the Ape Man's two-season series starring Ron Ely

Superman and the Jungle Devil (1953) and *Superman Flies Again* (1954): George Reeves as the Man of Steel in these three-segment pastiches

The Green Hornet (1974): assembled from the TV series in order to cash in on the popularity of martial-arts expert Bruce Lee, who co-starred as Kato

Zorro the Avenger (1960) and *The Sign of Zorro* (1960): theatrical editions of Walt Disney's TV hit

Davy Crockett, King of the Wild Frontier (1955) and *Davy Crockett and the Rover Pirates* (1956): three episodes each from the Disney TV program

Destination Alpha (1979): a pastiche of adventures from *Space: 1999*

The Forty-Eight Hour Mile (1970): a private-eye thriller constructed from two episodes of Darren McGavin's *The Outsider*

The celebrated star of the popular *My Three Sons* picks these as his favorites:

I Love Lucy
All in the Family
The Ed Sullivan Show ("Depending on who the guests were")
*M*A*S*H*
Barney Miller ("They have good people on it")

TV series which spawned big-budget theatrical films:

Get Smart, a popular spy spoof which ran from 1965–1969 gave birth to *The Nude Bomb* in 1980, with Don Adams repeating the role of Agent 86, Maxwell Smart.

Batman, the camp superhero program (1966–1968), was brought to the screen in the underrated, highly entertaining *Batman* (1966).

Star Trek, the borderline series which became a cult hit in syndication, inspired Paramount Pictures to lavish $43 million on a massive theatrical film in 1979. A sequel was recently released with a more modest budget of $10 million.

Head (1968), with the Monkees, whose TV series was a short-lived hit 1966–1967.

McHale's Navy and *McHale's Navy Joins the Air Force*, features released in 1964 and 1965 based on the successful (1962–1965) series

Munster, Go Home (1966), with the monsters seen in the 1964–1965 series.

The Muppet Movie (1979), featuring the puppet stars of the syndicated TV series, followed by *The Great Muppet Caper* two years later

What Do You Say to a Naked Lady? (1970), as Allen Funt takes his candid camera into situations far more risqué than he was permitted to do on the home screen

Changing the name of a series to disguise, improve, or indicate a cast overhaul:

The 20th Century became *The 21st Century,* looking from the present into the future, two-thirds way through its 1957–1969 run.

The Aquanauts (1960) became *Malibu Run* the second year, changing its emphasis from a *Sea Hunt* derivative to a *77 Sunset Strip* glamor-detective derivative.

The Little People (1972–1973) became *The Brian Keith Show.*

Meet Mr. McNutley became *The Ray Milland Show.*

All in the Family (1972–present) became *Archie Bunker's Place* three years ago.

Disneyland (1954–1980) changed regularly from *Disneyland* to *Walt Disney Presents* to *Walt Disney's Wonderful World of Color* to *The Wonderful World of Disney* to *Disney's Wonderful World.*

Mary (1978), Mary Tyler Moore's hour-long variety show, became *The Mary Tyler Moore Comedy Hour*, faring no better for it in 1979.

The Lucille Ball Show (1962–1973) became *The Lucy Show* and then *Here's Lucy.*

Battlestar Galactica (1978) was canceled and revived the following year as *Galactica 1980,* though its reincarnation with an all-new cast (save for paterfamilias Lorne Green) was short-lived.

The Pruitts of Southampton (1966) became *The Phyllis Diller Show.*

Burke's Law (1963–1965), starring Gene Barry as a flamboyant Los Angeles detective, became *Amos Burke: Secret Agent* in its final season, with the lawman going to work for the government.

Names of series characters . . . names which have become legend:

Archie Bunker (Carroll O'Connor) in *All in the Family* (1972–present)
Richard Kimble (David Janssen) in *The Fugitive* (1963–1966)
Matt Dillon (James Arness) in *Gunsmoke* (1955–1974)
Napoleon Solo (Robert Vaughn) in *The Man From U.N.C.L.E.* (1964–1967)
Sgt. Joe Friday (Jack Webb) in *Dragnet* (1952–1958 and 1967–1969)
Johnny Yuma (Nick Adams) in *The Rebel* (1959–1961)
Mr. Spock (Leonard Nimoy) in *Star Trek* (1966–1968)
Simon Templar (Roger Moore) in *The Saint* (1967–1968)
Inspector Lew Erskine (Efrem Zimbalist, Jr.) in *The F.B.I.* (1965–1973)
Kookie (Edd Byrnes) on *77 Sunset Strip* (more formally, Gerald Lloyd Kookson III) (1958–1963)
Ben Cartwright (Lorne Greene) of *Bonanza* (1959–1972)
Mike Nelson (Lloyd Bridges) in *Sea Hunt* (1958–1960)
Lucas McCain (Chuck Connors) in *The Rifleman* (1958–1962)
Cheyenne Bodie (Clint Walker) in *Cheyenne* (1955–1962)
Theo Kojak (Telly Savalas) in *Kojak* (1973-1977)

Col. Steve Austin (Lee Majors) *The 6 Million Dollar Man* (1974–1977)

Dr. Zorba (Sam Jaffe) in *Ben Casey* (1961–1965)

Maxwell Smart, Agent 86 (Don Adams), in *Get Smart* (1965–1969)

Fonzie (Henry Winkler) on *Happy Days* (1974–present) (officially, Arthur Fonzarelli)

Ralph Kramden (Jackie Gleason) on *The Honeymooners* (1955–1970)

Rob Petrie (Dick Van Dyke) on *The Dick Van Dyke Show* (1961–1965)

Each of these stars was noted for one hit show in particular—and was never able to recapture that glory in short-lived series which follows:

Vincent Edwards was a huge success as *Ben Casey* (1961–1965), yet his *Matt Lincoln* psychiatric portrayal perished early in 1971 after three months on the air.

Lorne Greene became a legend as Ben Cartwright on *Bonanza*, yet who remembers him as a private investigator in *Griff*, which vanished in January 1974 after three months.

David McCallum was a teen idol playing Illya Kuryakin on *The Man from U.N.C.L.E.* That show aired from 1964–1967. McCallum was considerably less fortunate playing a clandestine chap of a different sort: *The Invisible Man*, which premiered in September 1975 and itself became invisible the following January.

Sally Field, who became a TV celebrity as *The Flying Nun* (1967–1969), was unable to soar over bad ratings in her next series effort, *The Girl with Something Extra*, which ran from September of 1973 to May of 1974. Poor Ms. Field left TV for the movies, where she became a superstar and a best-actress Oscar-winner.

Robert Horton, who left *Wagon Train* after five years, vowed never to do another western. However, three years after leaving the popular series he was back in the saddle as *A Man Called Shenandoah* (1965), a victim of amnesia ("So roam/in search of home/cross this land so lonely," moaned the theme song—which he sang). The show was not a success.

Robert Conrad, closely identified with the part of superagent James T. West in *The Wild, Wild West* (1965–1969), has had a slew of series since then, from *The D.A.* to *A Man Called Sloane* to *Blacksheep Squadron.* None has worked, although Conrad is too formidable a player to count out yet.

William Shatner, whose career climbed as Capt. James Tiberius Kirk on *Star Trek* (1966–1968), was less lucky with *The Barbary Coast* (1975) as government agent Jeff Cable.

McLean Stevenson, after quitting the inordinately successful *M*A*S*H*, fell before the bull with *In the Beginning* (1978) and *The McLean Stevenson Show* (1976).

Bob Crane struck gold in *Hogan's Heroes* (1965–1970), then flopped in *The Bob Crane Show* (1975) prior to his tragic murder.

Andy Griffith, a giant in *The Andy Griffith Show* (1960–1967), failed to make tenure as *The Headmaster*, a high-school drama seen 1970–1971.

Roger Moore, who'd been immortalized as *The Saint*, could do nothing to assist Tony Curtis in *The Persuaders* (1971), abandoning TV in favor of film superstardom as the new James Bond.

Brian Keith, who had a surprise hit in *Family Affair* (1966–1970), was unable to find ratings harmony in *The Little People* or *Archer* (1975), and has gone back to motion pictures faring little better in flops like *Meteor* (1979) and *The Mountain Men* (1980). His best notices of late have come from starring in *Da* (1979) on Broadway.

Bobby Sherman, the singing sensation who starred in *Here Come the Brides* (1968–1969) and had a series of superhit recordings, managed to cripple his TV *and* singing career with the demise of *Getting Together* (1971).

Chuck Connors, the macho gun-toter in *The Rifleman,*

was a disgraced military officer in the far less successful western *Branded* (1965).

Phil Silvers' fondly remembered Sgt. Ernie Bilko of *The Phil Silvers Show* (1955–1958) was recycled as Harry Grafton in *The New Phil Silvers Show* (1963), but viewers didn't accept the comedian out of uniform.

Don Adams, who became one-and-the-same with Agent 86 on *Get Smart*, was a washout on *The Partners* (1971) as Detective Lennie Crooke.

Hard Sell

Movie and TV stars who have pitched products in TV commercials:

Vincent Price: Milton Bradley's game Hangman
Ernie Kovaks: Dutch Masters cigars
Steve Allen: Del Monte products
Laurence Olivier: Polaroid cameras
Joan Fontaine: Jove paperbacks
Frank Sinatra: Chrysler Motors
James Garner: Polaroid cameras
Bert Lahr: Lay's potato chips
Brenda Vaccaro: Playtex Tampons
O. J. Simpson: Hertz Rent-a-car
Bill Bixby: Dietac appetite suppressants
Ronald Reagan: Borax
Jack Klugman: Yogplait
Don Rickles and Lynda Carter: Diet 7-Up
Dick Van Patten: MVP diet powder
Ricardo Montalban: Chrysler Motors
Dinah Shore: Chevrolet
Bill Cosby: Jell-O
Sammy Davis, Jr.: Alka-Seltzer
John Houseman: Smith Barney, Harris Upham
Catherine Deneuve: Chanel
Ann Miller: Heinz's Great American Soups
Shirley Jones: Wesson oil
Louis Jourdan: Canada Dry club soda
Orson Welles: Paul Masson wine
Natalie Wood: Raintree moisturizer
Tony Randall: Prima Salsa tomato sauce
Karl Malden: American Express traveler's checks

Uncommon names used in the titles of TV series:

Szysznyk (1977): film star Ned Beatty portrayed the athletic director of a playground
Grindl (1963): Imogene Coca as an employee of a temporary-job service
Kaz (1978): Ron Leibman as attorney Kaz Kazinsky
Bronk (1975): movie heavy Jack Palance as Lt. Alexander Bronkov
Kojak: Telly Savalas as policeman Lt. Theo Kojak
Naika (1974): Deputy Sheriff Nakia Parker operating in the American southwest
Mannix (1967–1974): Mike Connors as Detective Joe Mannix
Kodiak (1974): Clint Walker as an Alaskan lawman who palled around with one Abraham Lincoln Imhook
Fish (1977): Detective Phil Fish from *Barney Miller* in his own sit com
O. K. Crackerby (1965): that's the full name of a billionaire, not an exclamatory adjective
Gomer Pyle, U.S.M.C. (1964–1969): the military man from Mayberry, North Carolina
Yancy Derringer (1958): Jock Mahoney as a New Orleans-based secret agent with an Indian chum by the name of Pahoo-Ka-Ta-Wah
The Kallilaks (1977): service station owners in Nowhere, California
Eischied (1979): a tough lawman

TV shows with initial impact:

M Squad (1957–1959)
The F.B.I. (1965–1973)
The Man from U.N.C.L.E. (1964–1967)
The Girl from U.N.C.L.E. (1966)
Mr. T & Tina
The Governor and J.J. (1969–1971)
W.E.B. (1978)
*M*A*S*H*
O. K. Crackerby
S.W.A.T. (1975)
Mayberry R.F.D. (1968–1970)
N.Y.P.D. (1967–1968)
Gomer Pyle, U.S.M.C.
T.H.E. Cat (1966–1967)
G.E. College Bowl (1968–1969)
U.S. Steel Hour (1953–1962)
The Robert Q. Lewis Show (1950)
Dr. I.Q. (1953)
MGM Parade (1955)
WKRP in Cincinnati (1978–present)
C.P.O. Sharkey (1976–1977)
Q.E.D. (1951)
Project U.F.O. (1978)
BJ and the Bear (1979–1980)
Trapper John, M.D. (1979–present)
Marcus Welby, M.D. (1969–1975)

Major U.S. cities which have served as the settings for TV series:

Philadelphia: *The Tony Randall Show* (1976–1977)
New York: *Kojak*
Los Angeles: *Lou Grant* (1977–present)
San Francisco: *Khan* (1975)
Dallas: *Dallas* (1978–present)
Washington, D.C.: *Grandpa Goes to Washington* (1978)
Las Vegas: *Blanskey's Beauties* (1977)
Honolulu: *Hawaii Five-O* (1968–1978)
Boston: *Beacon Hill* (1975)
Cincinnati: *WKRP in Cincinnati* (1978–present)
Chicago: Kolchak: *The Night Stalker* (1974)
Minneapolis: *The Mary Tyler Moore Show* (1970–1976)
Milwaukee: *Happy Days* (1974–present)
Phoenix: *Alice* (1976–present)
Miami: *Surfside Six* (1960–1961)
New Orleans: *Yancy Derringer* (1958)
Newark, New Jersey: *Toma* (1973)

Forget the exploitive show of the same name: these are people who, large or small, affected a large number of people:

Eliot Ness, played by Robert Stack on *The Untouchables* (1959–1962)
Daniel Boone, played by Fess Parker on *Daniel Boone* (1964–1969)
Wyatt Earp, played by Hugh O'Brian on *The Life and Legend of Wyatt Earp* (1955–1960)
Sir Francis Drake, played by Terence Morgan on *The Adventures of Sir Francis Drake* (1962)
Bat Masterson, played by Gene Barry on *Bat Masterson* (1959–1960)
Jim Bowie, played by Scott Forbes on *The Adventures of Jim Bowie* (1956–1957)
Jesse James, played by Christopher Jones on *The Legend of Jesse James* (1955–1965)
George Armstrong Custer, played by Wayne Maunder on *Custer* (1967)
Joy Adamson, played by Diana Muldaur on *Born Free* (1974)
Prince John, played by Ron Rifkin on *When Things Were Rotten* (1975)
General Lafayette, played by Philippe Forquet on *The Young Rebels* (1970)

The longest-running series in TV history:

Meet the Press: thirty-five seasons—still going strong
The Tonight Show: twenty-eight seasons, Mr. Carson hosting for twenty of those
Face the Nation: twenty-seven seasons
Disneyland (in its many versions): twenty-seven seasons, now defunct
The Lawrence Welk Show: twenty-seven seasons, the last ten in syndication
The Ed Sullivan Show: twenty-four seasons
The Cavalcade of Sports (Gillette): twenty-four seasons (originally local before network)
The Red Skelton Show: twenty seasons
Gunsmoke: twenty seasons (interestingly, the show was nearly dropped after its eleventh season, when there was a sudden surge in its popularity boosting it from the bottom of the ratings pack to the top ten)
What's My Line: eighteen seasons
Lassie: seventeen seasons
Kraft Television Theatre (in numerous guises): sixteen seasons
The Jack Benny Show: fifteen seasons
I've Got a Secret: fifteen seasons
The Honeymooners: fifteen seasons
Bonanza: fourteen seasons
The Adventures of Ozzie and Harriet: fourteen seasons
60 Minutes: thirteen seasons, still going strong
The Lucy Show: twelve seasons
My Three Sons: twelve seasons
The 20th Century (later, *The 21st Century*): twelve seasons
The Original Amateur Hour: twelve seasons

The longest-running series still on television:

Meet the Press: thirty-five seasons
The Tonight Show: twenty-eight seasons
Face the Nation: twenty-seven seasons
60 Minutes: thirteen seasons
All in the Family (also *Archie Bunker's Place*): eleven seasons
Monday Night Football: eleven seasons
*M*A*S*H*: ten seasons
Happy Days: eight seasons
Little House on the Prairie: eight seasons
Barney Miller: seven seasons
The Jeffersons: seven seasons
One Day at a Time: seven seasons
Laverne & Shirley: six seasons

Kings of the Hill

The top-rated individual TV shows in history:

1. *Dallas* ("Who Shot J.R.?")
2. *Roots* (Part Eight)
3. NBC's *Big Event* (*Gone With the Wind*, Part I)
4. *NBC Monday Night Movie* (*Gone With the Wind*, Part II)
5. Superbowl XII
6. Superbowl XIII
7. *Bob Hope Christmas Show* (1970)
8. *Roots* (Part Six)
9. *The Fugitive* (final episode, 8/29/67)
10. *Roots* (Part Five)
11. *Bob Hope Christmas Show* (1977)
12. *Roots* (Part Three)
13. *Ed Sullivan Show* (2/9/64, the Beatles)
14. Super Bowl XI
15. Super Bowl VI
16. *Roots* (Part Two)
17. *Beverly Hillbillies* (2/8/64)
18. *Roots* (Part Four)
19. Academy Awards (1964)
20. *Ed Sullivan Show* (1/15/64, the Beatles)
21. Super Bowl VII
22. Super Bowl IX
23. *Beverly Hillbillies* (2/26/64)
24. *Airport*
25. Super Bowl X
26. *Love Story*
27. *Cinderella*
28. *Roots* (Part Seven)
29. *Beverly Hillbillies* (3/25/64)
30. *Kickoff* (Super Bowl XII)

And the Winner Is . . .

Like the motion-picture industry, the television industry wasted little time creating an awards system to honor its own. The Emmy awards, an annual honor, are voted by TV professionals for their peers. The first Emmys were awarded in 1949, for programming aired during 1948. Among the winners in the awards' first few years are some legends, some who were ultimately losers, and some surprises:

Most Outstanding Personality (1952): Bishop Fulton J. Sheen
Best Actress (1952): Imogene Coca
Most Outstanding Kinescope (tape) Personality (1950): Milton Berle
Best Male Singer (1954): Perry Como
Best News Reporter (1954): John Daly
Best Audience Participation Series (1955): *The $64,000 Question* (later disgraced in a "cheating" scandal)
Most Outstanding Personality (1950): Groucho Marx
Best Single Program (1955): *Peter Pan*
Best Comedy Series (1957): *The Phil Silvers Show*
Best Actress in a Single Performance (1957): Polly Bergen in *The Helen Morgan Story* on *Playhouse 90*
Best Actor in a Single Performance (1956): Jack Palance in *Requiem for a Heavyweight* on *Playhouse 90*
Best Comedienne (1955): Nanette Fabray
Best Female Singer (1955): Dinah Shore
Best Public Affairs Program (1953): *Victory at Sea*
Best Live Show (1949): *The Ed Wynn Show*

Best Actor in a Regular Series (1954): Danny Thomas in *Make Room for Daddy*
Best Children's Program (1953): *Kukla, Fran & Ollie*
Best Performance by an Actor in a Continuing Role (1957): Robert Young in *Father Knows Best*
Best Performance by an Actress in a Continuing Role (1956): Loretta Young in *The Loretta Young Show*
Best Supporting Actress in a Dramatic Series (1958): Barbara Hale in *Perry Mason*
Best News Commentator (1958): Edward R. Murrow
Best Comedy Series (1958): *The Jack Benny Show*
Best Director, Live Series (1955): Franklin J. Schaffner, *The Caine Mutiny Court-Martial* on *Ford Star Jubilee* (Schaffner went on to become a theatrical director, helming such films as *Patton* and *Planet of the Apes*)
Best Producer (1955): Walt Disney
Best Teleplay (1957): Rod Serling, *The Comedian*, on *Playhouse 90* (one of Serling's many Emmy awards)
Best News Series (1958): *The Huntley-Brinkley Report*
Best Western Series (1958): *Maverick* (there were so many westerns that the genre required its own category)
Best Actor in a Series (1959): Robert Stack for *The Untouchables*
Best Single Performance by an Actress (1959): Ingrid Bergman in *The Turn of the Screw* on *Ford Startime*
Best Television Personality (1948): Shirley Dinsdale and Judy Splinters (her puppet)

Cardinal TV

Programs with numbers in their title, both cardinal and ordinal:

90 Bristol Court (1964)
Adam 12 (1968–1974)
Room 222 (1969–1973)
Space: 1999 (1976–1977)
60 Minutes (1968–present)
6 Million Dollar Man (1974–1978)
Hawaii Five-O (1968–1979)
77 Sunset Strip (1958–1963)
Ball Four (1976)
The Second Hundred Years (1967)
Route 66 (1960–1963)
Car 54, Where Are You? (1961–1962)
Surfside Six
Colt .45 (1957–1959)
Playhouse 90 (1956–1960)
Two for the Money (1952–1957)
Tales of the 77th Bengal Lancers (1956)
Cain's Hundred (1961)
Studio 57 (1954)
Twenty-One (1956–1957)
Twenty Questions (1949–1954)
20/20 (1978–present)
20th Century (1957–1969) (because *21st Century* in 1967)
My Three Sons (1960–1971)
Paris 7000 (1970)
240 Robert (1979)
Eight Is Enough (1977–present)
Nashville 99 (1977)

Almost every program on the air originates as a one-shot sample program or "pilot." If it looks like a stinker, the show never gets beyond that stage. Here are pilots which were produced but never made it to the air:

Richard the Lionhearted (1956) and *The Three Musketeers* (1956) both of these produced during the medieval craze which gave us *Robin Hood, Ivanhoe, Sir Lancelot*, and others

Return to Peyton Place (1979), a videotaped prime-time soaper

The Sheriff's Wife (1957)

Fremont the Trailblazer (1957)

Tales of the Vikings (1959), based on the 1958 Kirk Douglas film

Alexander the Great (1966), starring William Shatner

Hercules (1965), starring muscleman and former movie Tarzan Gordon Scott in one of the most expensive pilots in TV history

Ghostbreaker (1965), starring Kerwin Mathews as a traveling exorcist

Alfred of the Amazon (1966), a Tarzan spoof

Tar Gar (1966), a jungle hero played by ex-Tarzan Mike Henry

Superboy (1960), an attempt to cash in on the successful *Superman* TV series

The Magic of Sinbad (1960), starring Lassie's ex-boss Tommy Retig

The Barbarians (1960), with Jack Palance as Rivak, warrior of the Punic Wars

Lafitte the Pirate (1960), starring Fernando Lamas

Hercule Poirot (1960), featuring José Ferrer as Agatha Christie's immortal detective
Boston Terrier (1960), produced by Blake Edwards (of *Pink Panther* and *10* fame) and starring Robert Vaughn as the foppish sleuth
Mandrake the Magician (1966), based on the comic strip, and remade as a TV movie in 1980
Mr. Zero (1967), about an alien who comes to earth to abolish evil
Nuts & Bolts (1981), starring Rich Little as a robot manufacturer
In Trouble (1981), about three girls who work as barmaids
Rise and Shine (1981), the doings at a co-ed boarding school

Many continuing characters are known primarily by their last names. Here are some of the obscure first names of such personalities:

Family (1976–1978): "Buddy" Lawrence (Kristy McNichol) was Letitia

Family Affair: Mr. French (Sebastian Cabot) was Giles

Voyage to the Bottom of the Sea: Admiral Nelson (Richard Basehart) was Harriman

The Man from U.N.C.L.E.: Mr. Waverly (Leo G. Carroll) was Alexander

Kung Fu (1972–1974): Caine (David Carradine) was Kwai Chang

Gunsmoke (1955–1974): Doc Adams (Milburn Stone) was Galen

Star Trek: Ensign Chekov (Walter Koenig) was Pavel

Get Smart: The Chief (Edward Platt) was Thaddeus

Mr. Peepers (1965): Mr. Peepers (Wally Cox) was Robinson

Mr. Novak (1963–1964): Mr. Novak (James Franciscus) was John

Judd, for the Defense (1967–1968): Judd (Carl Betz) was Clinton

Kojak: Kojak (Telly Savalas) was Theo

Dennis the Menace (1959–1962): Mr. Wilson (Joseph Kearns/Gale Gordon) was George

Dr. Kildare (1961–1965): Dr. Kildare (Richard Chamberlain) was James

Dr. Kildare: Dr. Gillespie (Raymond Massey) was Leonard

I'm Dickens—He's Fenster (1962): Fenster (Marty Ingels) was Arch

I'm Dickens—He's Fenster: Dickens (John Astin) was Harry
Shaft: Shaft (Richard Roundtree) was John
Fish: Detective Fish (Abe Vigoda) was Phil
The Famous Adventures of Mr. Magoo: Mr. Magoo (Jim Backus, voice) was Quincy

TV characters and their places of employment:

Fred Flintstone (*The Flintstones*): The Rock Head and Quarry Cave Construction Co.
Arnie Nuvo (*Arnie*): The Continental Flange Co.
Laverne De Fazio and Shirley Feeney (*Laverne & Shirley*): The Shotz Brewery
Archie Bunker (*All in the Family*): Prendergast Tool and Die Company
Walter Findlay (*Maude*): Findlay's Friendly Appliances
Dr. Ben Casey (*Ben Casey*): County General Hospital
Dr. James Kildare (*Dr. Kildare*): Blair General Hospital
Britt Reid (*The Green Hornet*): *The Daily Sentinel*
Bill Davis (*Family Affair*): consulting engineer
Darrin Stephens (*Bewitched*): The Tate & Mann Advertising Agency
Phyllis Lindstrom (*Phyllis*): Erskine's Commercial Photography Studio
Joe Gerard (*Rhoda*): The New York Wrecking Company
Mary Richards (*The Mary Tyler Moore Show*): WJM-TV
Lou Grant (*Lou Grant*): *The Los Angeles Tribune*
Gabe Kotter (*Welcome Back, Kotter*): James Buchanan High School
Ann Romano (*One Day at a Time*): The Connors & Davenport Advertising Agency
Dick Smothers (*The Smothers Brothers Show*): Pandora Publishing Company
Tom Bradford (*Eight Is Enough*): *The Sacramento* (California) *Register*

Doris Martin (*The Doris Day Show*): *Today's World* magazine
Alice Hyatt (*Alice*): Mel's Diner
Herman Munster (*The Munsters*): The Gateman, Goodbury & Graves Funeral Home
Tim O'Hara (*My Favorite Martian*): *The Los Angeles Sun*
Carl Kolchak (*Kolchak: The Night Stalker*): The Independent News Service
Connie Brooks (*Our Miss Brooks*): Madison High School
Seymour Kaufman (*Room 222*): Walt Whitman High School
James Nash (*Please Don't Eat the Daisies*): Ridgemont College
Rob Petrie (*The Dick Van Dyke Show*): *The Alan Brady Show*
Susanna Pomeroy (*The Gale Storm Show*): The SS Ocean Queen (social director)
Porter Ricks (*Flipper*): Coral Key Park (Florida)
Jim Anderson (*Father Knows Best*): General Insurance Company
Gunther Toody (*Car 54, Where Are You?*): 53rd Precinct (New York)
Barney Miller (*Barney Miller*): 12th Precinct
Oscar Madison (*The Odd Couple*): *The New York Herald*

Famous composers of TV scores and/or famous scores by little-known composers:

Mission: Impossible: Lalo Schifrin
Batman: Neil Hefti
Battlestar Galactica; Buck Rogers: Stu Phillips
Maya: Hans J. Salter
Perry Mason: Fred Steiner
Kolchak: the Night Stalker; *Night Gallery*: Gil Melle
The Prisoner: Ron Grainer
Star Trek (theme): Alexander Courage
Thriller; *The Loner*: Jerry Goldsmith
Twilight Zone (theme): Bernard Herrmann
Mr. Lucky; *Peter Gunn*: Henry Mancini
Combat; *The Defenders*; *Marcus Welby, M.D.*: Leonard Rosenman
The Outer Limits; *One Step Beyond*: Henry Lubin
Lost In Space; *The Time Tunnel*; *Land of the Giants*: Johnny Williams
I Love Lucy: Wilbur Hatch
Victory at Sea: Richard Rogers
The F.B.I.: Bronislau Kaper

TV shows based on comic strips or comic books (live action):

The Adventures of Superman (1951–1956): comic book
Blondie: comic strip (1957), (1968)
Batman: comic book
Dick Tracy (1950): comic strip
Wonder Woman (1976–1978): comic book
The Incredible Hulk (1978–1980): comic book
Spiderman (1978): comic book
Lost in Space (1965–1967): comic book entitled *Space Family Robinson*
Hazel (1961–1965): comic strip
Dennis the Menace: comic-panel character
The Addams Family (1964–1965): comic-panel characters
Steve Canyon (1958–1959): comic strip

Walt Disney was one of the few Hollywood producers who was unafraid of television when it began to cut into theatrical receipts in the early 1950s. He saw the medium as an outlet for product old and new, and for a means of *promoting* his theatrical features, as well as his new amusement park Disneyland. However commercial his motives, Disney nonetheless made a lasting contribution to the tube. His series and some of their legendary miniseries are listed below:

Disneyland (1954–present): under various names, the hour-long show presented, weekly, adventures, cartoons, science programs, and serials; among the latter were such popular characters as:
- *Elfego Baca*, played by Robert Loggia, a frontier lawman ("And the legend was that, like el Gato, the Cat, nine lives had Elfego Baca")
- *Texas John Slaughter*, starring Tom Tryon as a crack-shot lawman
- *The Saga of Andy Burnett*, Jerome Courtland as a mountain man
- *Swamp Fox*, being the exploits of Revolutionary War hero Francis Marion, played by Leslie Nielsen
- *Davy Crockett*, the one-and-only legendary fad starring Fess Parker

The Mickey Mouse Club (1955–1958): the most polished of all children's programs, featuring such classic serials as:
- *The Hardy Boys*
- *Corky and White Shadow*
- *Spin and Marty*
- *The Boys of the Western Sea*

Zorro (1957–1958): Guy Williams as the masked avenger of old California, and another fad-setter

The Mouse Factory: Disney's ill-fated experiment in the 1970s at syndicating a show constructed around Disney cartoons, with a variety of guest hosts

The New Mickey Mouse Club (1975–1976): short-lived and strained, showing that the great idea had been supplanted by greater ideas

Specials: Over the years, Disney feature films have been aired as NBC movies; among them, *Twenty Thousand Leagues Under the Sea* and *Dumbo*

Animated Opening

Live-action series which used cartoon animation for the opening titles:

I Dream of Jeannie (1965–1969)
The Smothers Brothers Show (1965)
Batman
Mr. Terrific (1967)
Lost in Space (1965–1967)
The Carol Burnett Show (1967–1977)
The Partridge Family (1970–1973)
Bewitched (1964–1971)
Disneyland
Fractured Flickers (1963)

Husband-and-wife acting teams in TV, past and present:

Heather Menzies (*Logan's Run*) and Robert Urich (*Vegas*)
Gil Gerard (*Buck Rogers*) and Connie Sellecca (*The Greatest American Hero*)
Lee Majors (*The Six Million Dollar Man*) and Farrah Fawcett (*Charlie's Angels*)
Dennis Cole (*The Felony Squad*) and Jaclyn Smith (*Charlie's Angels*)
Lucille Ball and Desi Arnaz (*I Love Lucy*)
Shirley Jones (*The Partridge Family*) and Jack Cassidy (*He & She*)
Paula Prentiss and Richard Benjamin (*He & She*)
John Astin (*The Addams Family*) and Patty Duke (*The Patty Duke Show*)
Sonny and Cher (*The Sonny and Cher Comedy Hour*)
George Burns and Gracie Allen (*The George Burns and Gracie Allen Show*)
Martin Landau and Barbara Bain (*Mission: Impossible* and *Space: 1999*)
David Birney and Meredith Baxter (*Bridget Loves Bernie*)
Valerie Harper (*Rhoda*) and Richard Schaal (*Phyllis*)
Ozzie Nelson and Harriet Nelson (*The Adventures of Ozzie and Harriet*)
Jack Klugman and Brett Somers (*The Odd Couple*)
Christopher George (*The Rat Patrol*) and Lynda Day George (*Mission: Impossible*)

Other than husband and wife, there are various kinfolk who've worked on TV:

Jock Mahoney (*Yancy Derringer*) is stepfather to Sally Field (*The Flying Nun*).
Tom and Dick Smothers (*The Smothers Brothers Show*) are, of course, brothers.
James Arness (*Gunsmoke*) and Peter Graves (*Mission: Impossible*) are brothers.
George C. Scott (*East Side/West Side*) and Devon Scott (*The Tony Randall Show*) are father and daughter.
Danny Thomas (*Make Room for Daddy*) is father to Marlo Thomas (*That Girl*).
Helen Hayes (*The Snoop Sisters*) is the mother of James MacArthur (*Hawaii Five-O*).
Beau Bridges (*Ensign O'Toole*) is the son of Lloyd Bridges (*Sea Hunt*).
Sean Cassidy (*The Hardy Boys*) is brother to David Cassidy (*The Partridge Family*), both sons to the late Jack Cassidy (*He & She*).
Paula Prentiss (*He & She*) is the sister of Ann Prentiss (*Captain Nice*).
Dick Van Dyke (*The Dick Van Dyke Show*) is the brother of Jerry Van Dyke (*My Mother the Car*).
Rob Reiner (*All in the Family*) is the son of Carl Reiner (*The Dick Van Dyke Show*).
John Carradine (*My Friend Irma*) is the father of David Carradine (*Kung Fu*).

Take a Hike

Stars who have walked off or otherwise departed hit series:

Clayton Moore from *The Lone Ranger* (1949–1956), replaced for two seasons by John Hart

Erik Estrada from *CHiPS* (1977–present), at the beginning of the 1981 season

Lynn Redgrave from *House Calls* (1979–present), ostensibly when Universal Studios failed to make accommodations for her to breast-feed her baby; the studio claims salary was the real dispute

Suzanne Somers from *Three's Company* (1977–present), over a salary dispute at the end of the 1980 season

James Garner from *Maverick* (1957–1961), in 1960 over a contract dispute; he is back, now, in a revival of the series

Clint Walker from *Cheyenne* (1955–1962) for 1958–1959, over the split of subsidiary rights from the show

Richard Thomas from *The Waltons* (1972–present), looking to expand his career beyond the series; moving to Broadway, he drew better notices than Christopher Reeve in *The Fifth of July*

Johnny Carson from *The Tonight Show Starring Johnny Carson* (1962–present), in a salary snag

Diana Rigg from *The Avengers* (1966–1968), to pursue other interests in 1968, although program execs said that, anyway, they *wanted* a younger, sexier co-star. Sexier?!

Dick York from *Bewitched* in 1969, replaced by Dick Sargent

Steven Hill starred in *Mission: Impossible* (1966–

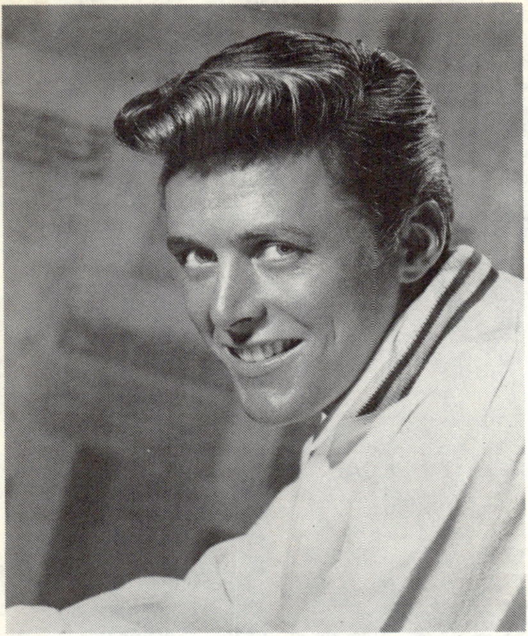

77 Sunset Strip (see *HISTORIC HANDLES*, page *25*)

Buck Rogers in the 25th Century (see *RERUNS*, page *16*)
© *NBC TV*

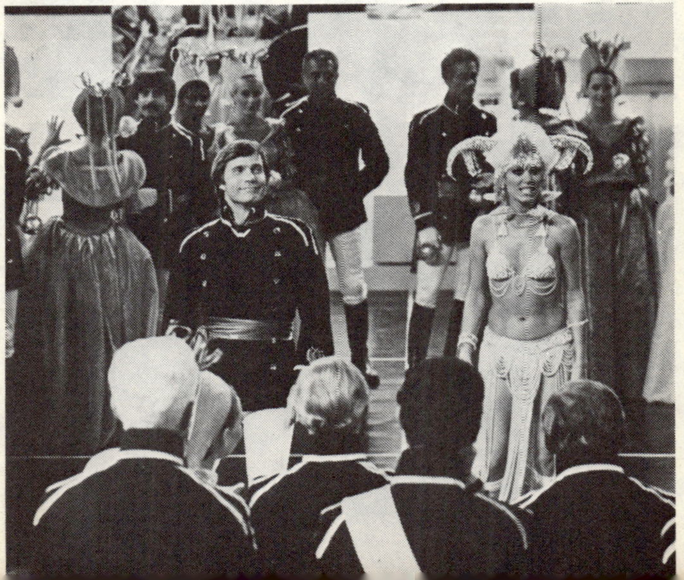

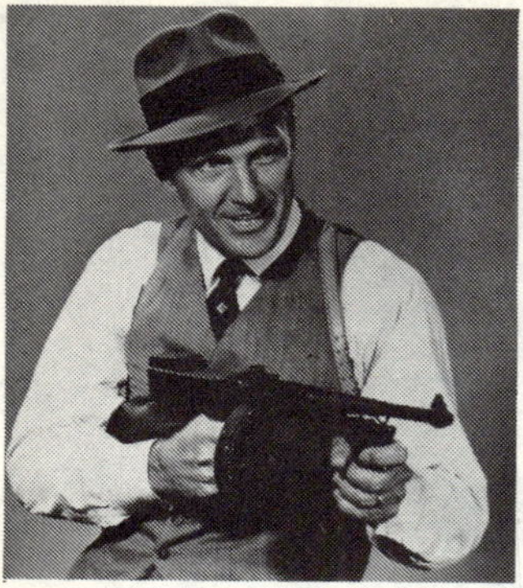

The Untouchables (see *REAL PEOPLE*, page *34*)

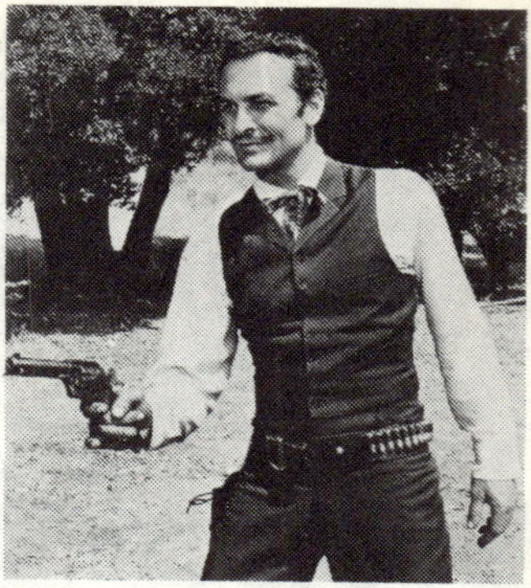

Elfego Baca (see *WALT'S LEGACY*, page *49*) © *Walt Disney Productions*

The Rifleman (see *HISTORIC HANDLES*, page *25*)

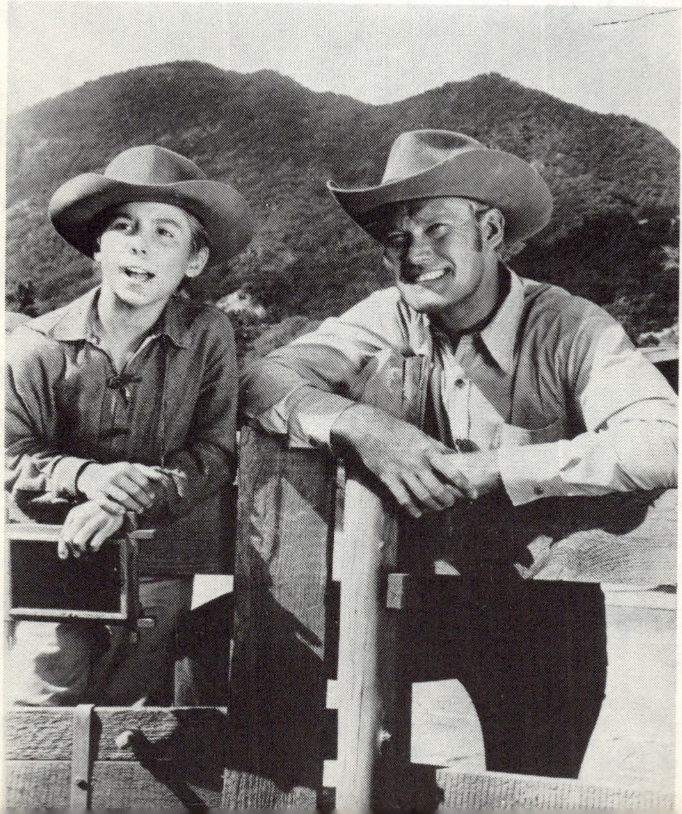

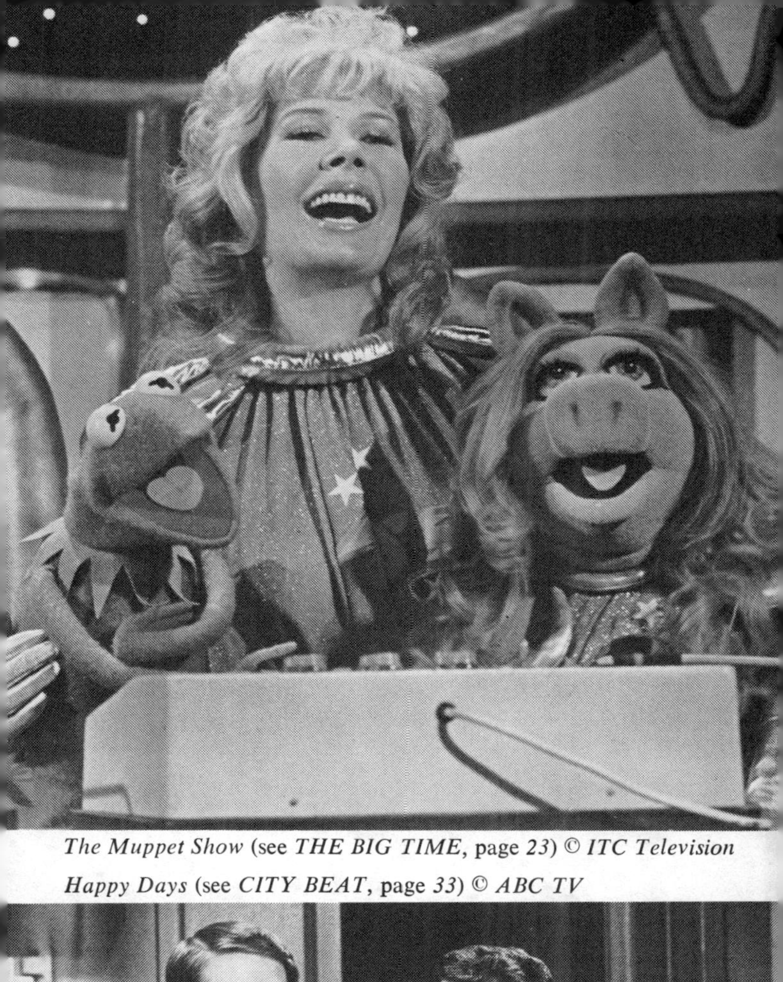

The Muppet Show (see *THE BIG TIME*, page *23*) © *ITC Television*

Happy Days (see *CITY BEAT*, page *33*) © *ABC TV*

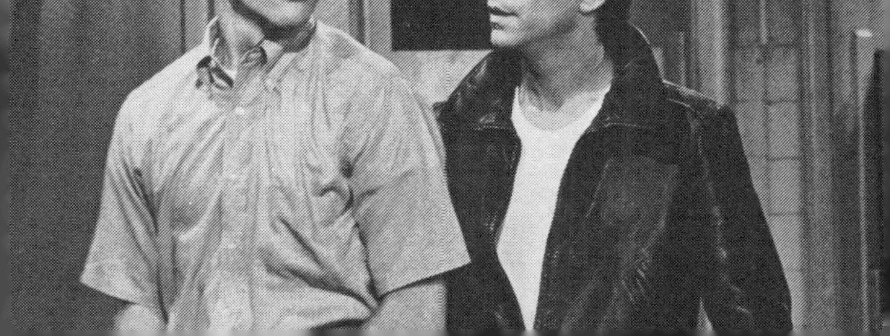

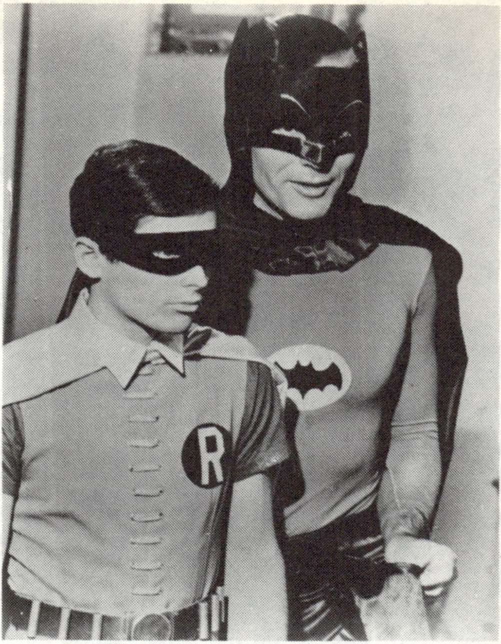

Batman (see *THE BIG TIME*, page *23*)

The 6 Million Dollar Man (see *QUITE A CHARACTER*, page *62*)

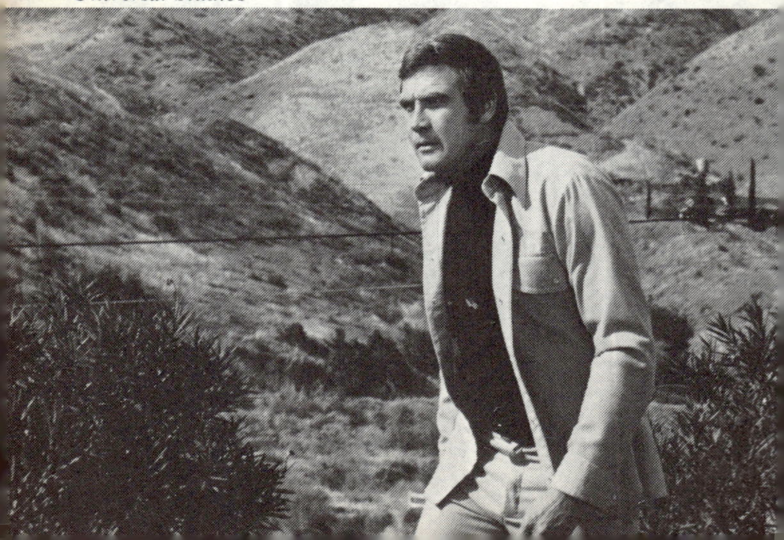

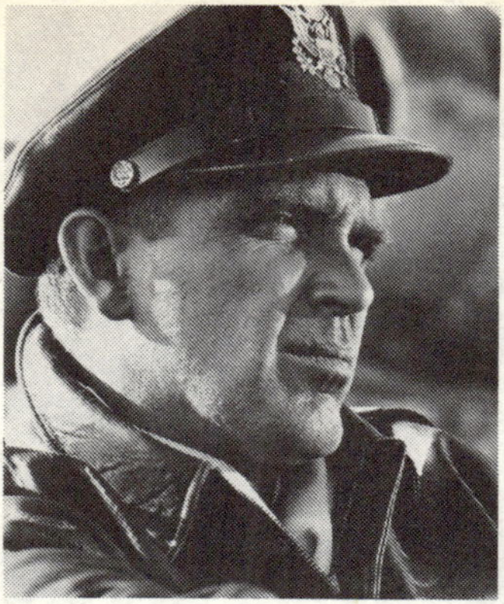

Twelve O'Clock High (see *TO BE CONTINUED*, page *6*) © *20th Century-Fox Television*

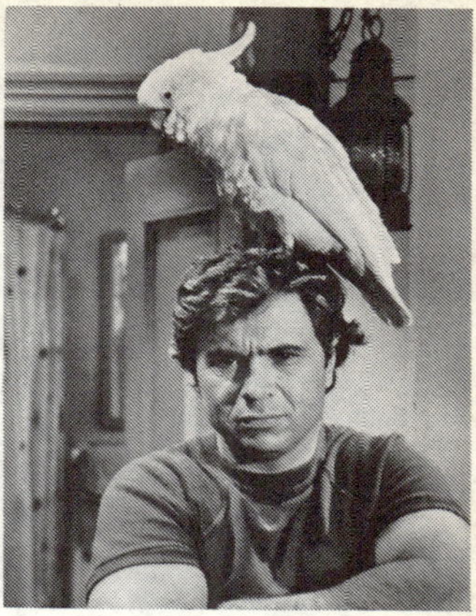

Baretta (see *WHAT'S IN A NAME*, page *68*) © *ABC TV*

Ross Martin in *The Wild, Wild West* (*DEDICATION*)

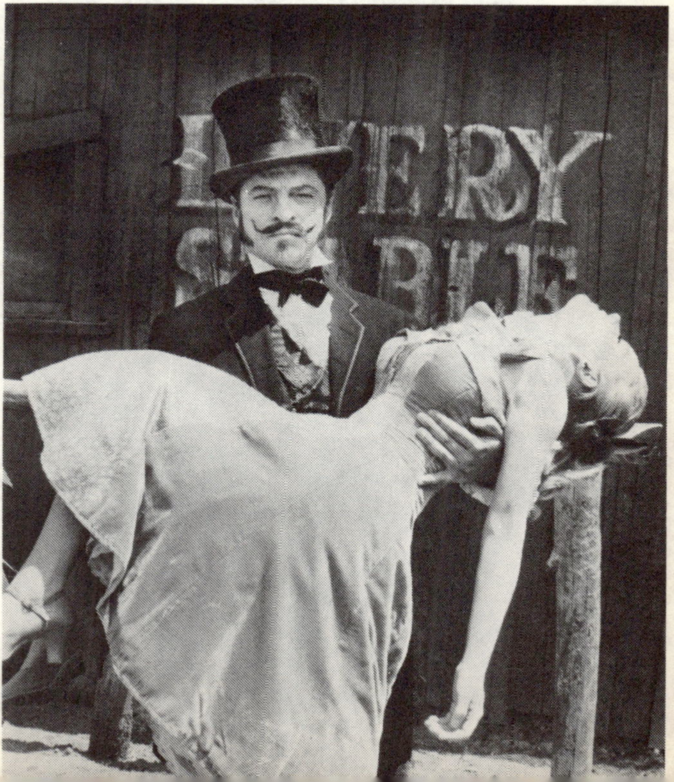

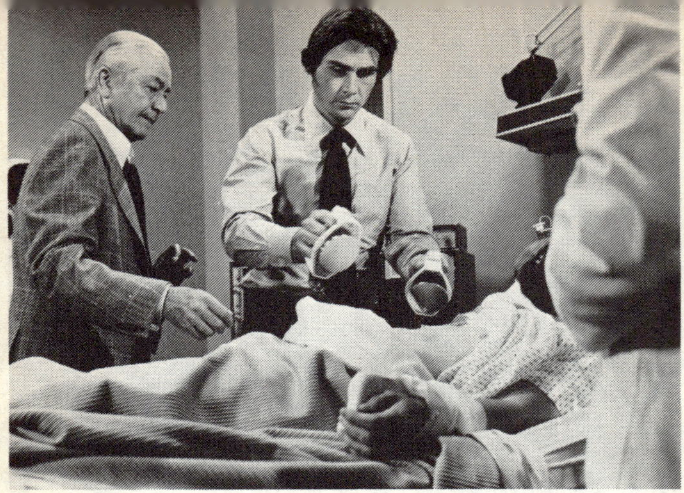

Marcus Welby, M.D. (see *LIGHTNING STRIKES TWICE*, page *67*) © *ABC TV*

Ironside (see *LIGHTNING STRIKES TWICE*, page *66*)

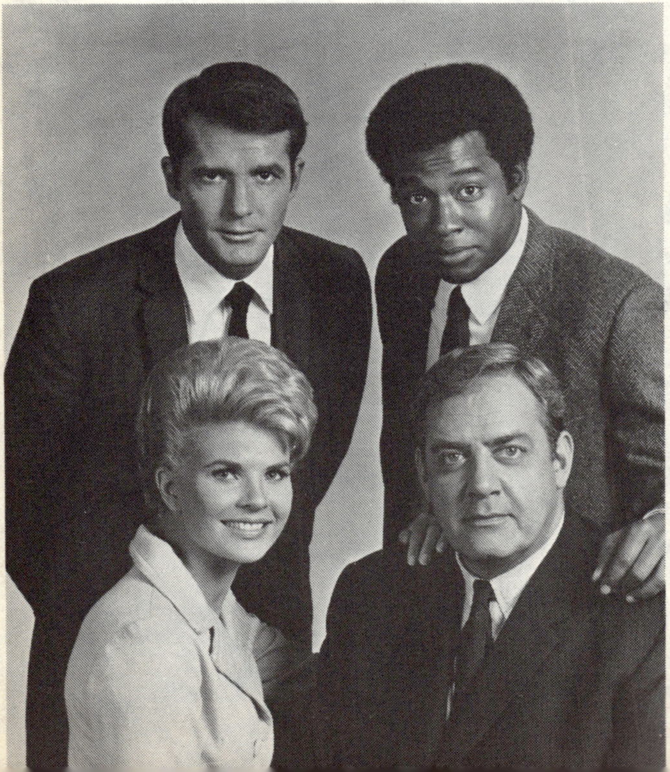

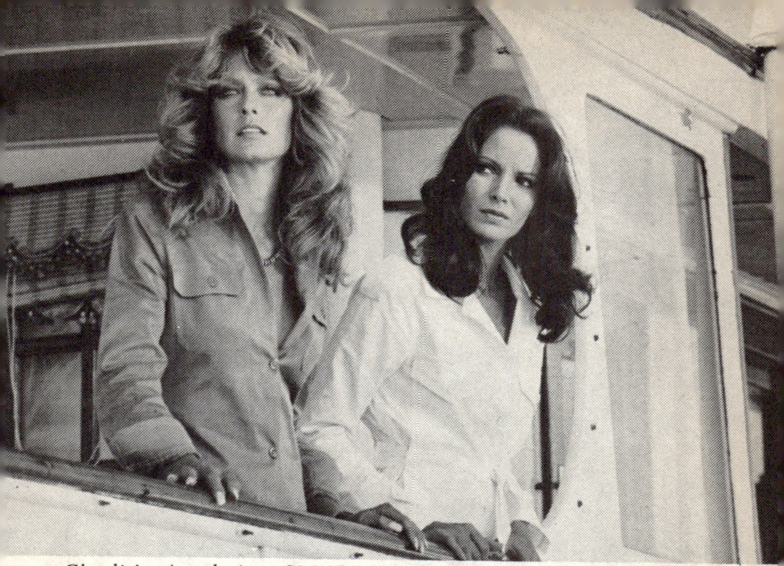

Charlie's Angels (see *SMALL-TIME BLOCKBUSTERS*, page *81*)

Davy Crockett (see *SPLICE OF LIFE*, page *21*)
© *Walt Disney Productions*

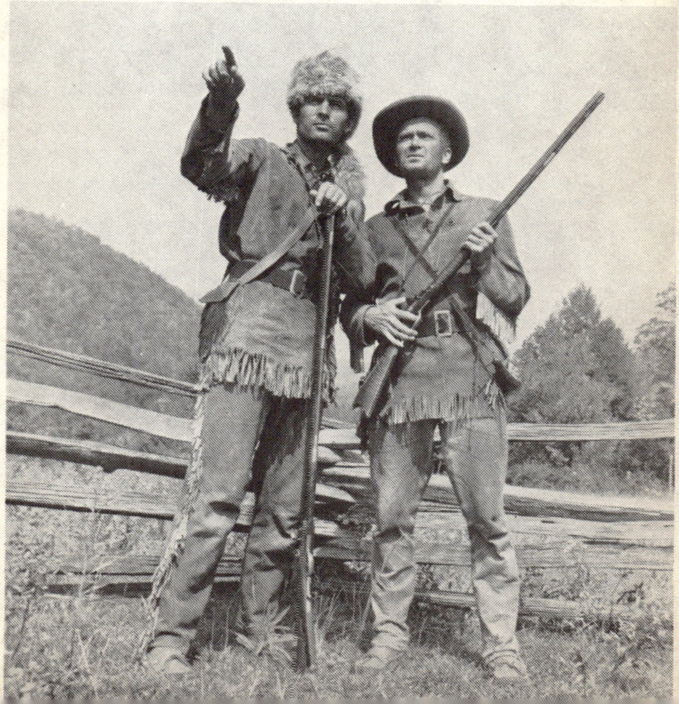

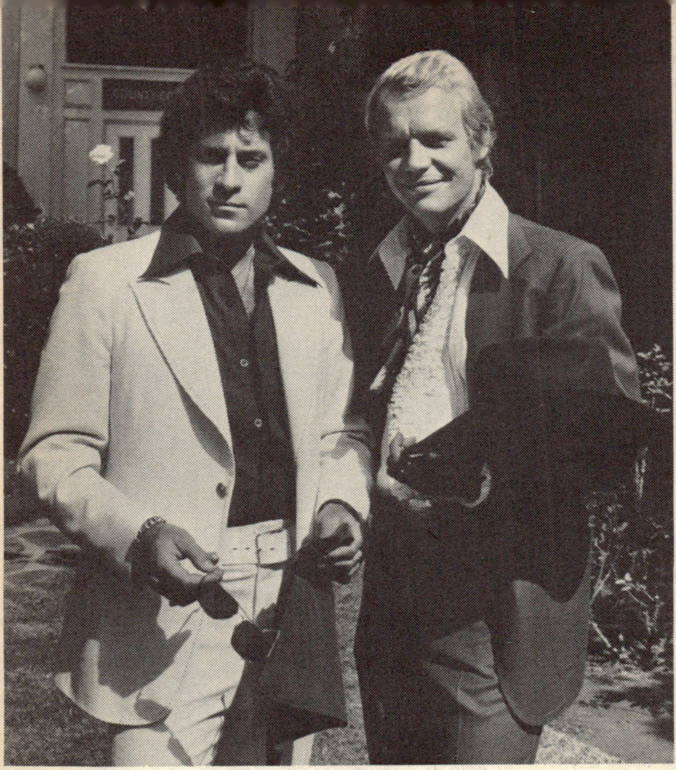

Starsky and Hutch (see *TEAMWORK*, page *10*) © *ABC TV*

Tarzan's Deadly Silence (see *SPLICE OF LIFE*, page *21*) © *NBC Television*

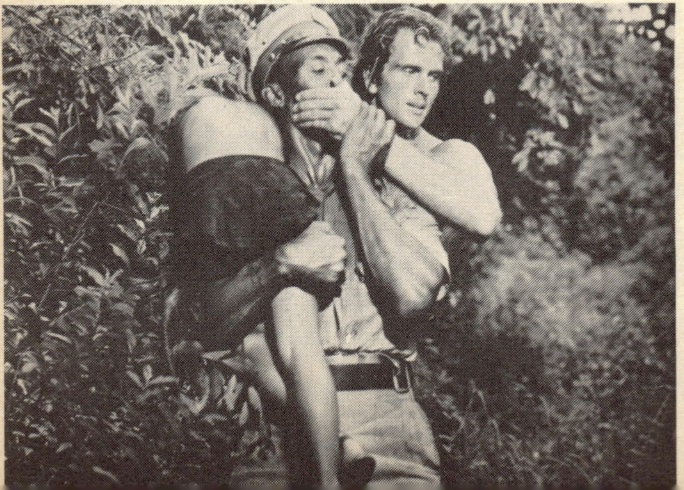

1972) for the first of its six seasons; he is said to have left when they refused to close down shooting by Friday evenings, when he celebrated the commencement of the Sabbath. Peter Graves took over

Wayne Rogers, since leaving *M*A*S*H*, has fared far better than many of his fellow evacuees such as McLean Stevenson, Gary Burghoff, and Larry Linville: he has diversified by starring in, among other shows, the current hit *House Calls*

The longest titles of continuing TV series (tallied by characters sans spaces):

1. *Kraft Music Hall Presents the Des O'Connor Show*
2. *Lawrence Welk's Top Tunes and New Talent Show*
3. *The Ford Show Starring Tennessee Ernie Ford*
4. *The All-American Football Game of the Week*
5. *James Michener's Adventures in Paradise*
6. *The Tonight Show Starring Johnny Carson*
7. *Walt Disney's Wonderful World of Color*
8. *The Tony Orlando and Dawn Rainbow Hour*
9. *Bob Hope Presents the Chrysler Theatre*
10. *The George Burns and Gracie Allen Show*
11. *Lawrence Welk's Dodge Dancing Party*
12. *The Adventures of Ozzie and Harriet*
13. *The Smothers Brothers Comedy Hour*
14. *The Life and Times of Grizzly Adams*
15. *The Famous Adventures of Mr. Magoo*
16. *The New Adventures of Wonder Woman*
17. *The Travels of Jaimie McPheeters*
18. *The Roy Rogers and Dale Evans Show*
19. *Sammy Kaye's Music from Manhattan*
20. *The Life and Legend of Wyatt Earp*
21. *The Mary Tyler Moore Comedy Hour*
22. *The NBC Wednesday Mystery Movie*
23. *Dick Powell's Zane Grey Theatre*
24. *Perry Como's Kraft Music Hall*
25. *The Many Loves of Dobie Gillis*
26. *Voyage to the Bottom of the Sea*

Company or product names that were actually a *part* of a TV series' title:

Gillette Cavalcade of Sports
Philco TV Playhouse
Kraft Television Theatre
G.E. College Bowl
Chesterfield Supper Club
Ford Theatre
Colgate Comedy Hour
Schlitz Playhouse of Stars
Pabst Blue Ribbon Bouts
Armstrong Circle Theatre
Gulf Playhouse
Texaco Star Theatre (*The Milton Berle Show*)
U.S. Steel Hour
Motorola TV Theatre
Goodyear TV Playhouse
Campbell Soundstage
Buick Berle Show
Alcoa Hour
Voice of Firestone
DuPont Theatre
Dinah Shore Chevy Show
Lux Playhouse
Bell Telephone Hour
Bob Hope Presents the Chrysler Theatre

Actresses who have played supporting-character, TV mothers:

Barbara Eden as both Jeannie and Jeannie's mother on *I Dream of Jeannie* (1965–1969)
Nancy Walker as Ida Morgenstern on *Rhoda* (1974–1978)
Jean Byron as Natalie on *The Patty Duke Show* (1963–1965)
Agness Moorehead as Endora on *Bewitched*
Cloris Leachman/June Lockhart as Ruth Martin on *Lassie* (1954–1970)
Barbara Billingsley as June Cleaver on *Leave it to Beaver* (1957–1962)
Gloria Henry as Alice Mitchell on *Dennis the Menace*
Alice Ghostley as Mrs. Nash on *Captain Nice* (1967)
Marion Ross as Marion Cunningham on *Happy Days*
Rosemary DeCamp as Helen Marie on *That Girl* (1966–1970)
Jane Wyatt as Margaret Anderson on *Father Knows Best* (1954–1962)
Marjorie Lord as Kathy Williams on *The Danny Thomas Show* (1953–1964)
Audra Lindley as Amy Fitzgerald on *Bridget Loves Bernie* (1972)
Florence Henderson as Carol Brady on *The Brady Bunch* (1969–1973)
Cloris Leachman as Queen Hippolyte on *Wonder Woman*
Shirley Jones as Connie Partridge on *The Partridge Family* (1970–1973)

. . . and a few daughters:

Christine Matchett as Melissa Marshall on *Owen Marshall, Counselor at Law* (1971–1973)
Diane and Erin Murphy as Tabitha Stephens on *Bewitched* (1964–1971)
Devon Scott (daughter of George C.)/Penny Peyser as Roberta Franklin on *The Tony Randall Show* (1976–1977)
Angela Powell as Annie Preston on *The New Dick Van Dyke Show* (1971–1973)
Adrienne Barbeau as Carol on *Maude* (1972–1977)
Veronica Cartwright as Jemima Boone on *Daniel Boone* (1964–1969)
Angela Cartwright as Penny Robinson on *Lost in Space* (1965–1967)
Jodie Foster as Elizabeth Henderson on *Bob & Carol & Ted & Alice* (1973)

Keep the Faith

Holy people who have been regular characters in TV series:

Rev. Tom Holvak (Glenn Ford) *The Family Holvak* (1975–1976)
Father John Mulcahy (William Christopher) *M*A*S*H* (1977)
Rabbi David Small (Bruce Solomon) *Lanigan's Rabbi* (1977)
Father Daniel M. Cleary (McLean Stevenson) *In the Beginning* (1978)
Father Chuck O'Malley (Gene Kelly) *Going My Way* (1962)
Father Fitzgibbon (Leo G. Carroll) *Going My Way* (1962)
Sister Bertrille (Sally Field) *The Flying Nun* (1967–1969)
Mother Superior (Madeleine Sherwood) *The Flying Nun* (1967–1969)
Father Mike Fitzgerald (Robert Sampson) *Bridget Loves Bernie* (1972)
Friar Tuck (Alexander Gauge) *The Adventures of Robin Hood* (1955–1957)
Friar Tuck (Dick Van Patten) *When Things Were Rotten* (1975)
Rev. Tom Winter (Bob Hogan) *Peyton Place* (1964–1968)

Quite a Character

Some of the more unusual continuing roles undertaken by actors in television series:

Ann Sothern as a 1928 Porter in *My Mother the Car* (1965)
Julie Newmar as a robot in *My Living Doll* (1964)
Barbara Eden as a genie in *I Dream of Jeannie* (1965–1969)
Leonard Nimoy as an emotionless alien in *Star Trek* (1966–1968)
Adam West as a costumed crimefighter-millionaire in *Batman*
Ron Ely as a man raised by apes in *Tarzan* (1966–1968)
Sally Field as an airborne convent-dweller in *The Flying Nun*
Sally Field, this time as a psychic in *The Girl with Something Extra* (1973)
Peter Kastner as a woman in *The Ugliest Girl in Town* (1968)
George Reeves as a superbeing from another world in *The Adventures of Superman* (1951–1957)
Mary Jane Croft as the voice of the dog Cleo in *The People's Choice* (1955–1957)
Imogene Coca as a cave woman in *It's About Time* (1966)
James Darren as a man who floats through time in *The Time Tunnel* (1966)
Tommy Smothers as an angel in *The Smothers Brothers Show* (1965)
Andy Christopher as a devil in *Mr. Black* (1949)
Marshall Thompson as a six-inch-tall secret agent in *World of Giants* (1959)

Edward Mulhare as a specter in *The Ghost and Mrs. Muir* (1968–1969)

Roddy McDowall as an articulate chimpanzee in *Planet of the Apes* (1974)

Lee Majors as a half-man, half-machine in *The 6 Million Dollar Man* (1974–1977)

Monte Markham as a prospector, thawed from glaciation after sixty-seven years in *The Second Hundred Years* (1967)

Ray Walston as a denizen of the fourth planet in *My Favorite Martian* (1963–1965)

David McCallum as a transparent scientist in *The Invisible Man* (1975)

Christopher Geroge as a man who is unable to die in *The Immortal* (1970)

Elizabeth Montgomery as a sorceress in *Bewitched*

Al Lewis as a vampire in *The Munsters* (1964–1965), which also featured Fred Gwynn as the Frankenstein Monster

Catherine Schell as a shape-changing alien in *Space: 1999* (1976–1977)

Richard Kelton as Ficus, the planet man of *Quark* (1978)

Motion-picture superstars who did early work in television series:

- Burt Reynolds as *Dan August* (1970) and *Hawk* (1966)
- Charles Bronson in *Man with a Camera* (1958–1959) as Mike Kovac
- Clint Eastwood in *Rawhide* (1959–1965) as Rowdy Yates
- John Travolta in *Welcome Back, Kotter* (1975–1978)
- Christopher Reeve in *Love of Life* (an ongoing role which he played in the soap opera before becoming *Superman*)
- Jack Lemmon in the sit com *Heaven for Betsy* (1952)
- Ryan O'Neal as Rodney Harrington on *Peyton Place* (1964–1968)
- Richard Dreyfuss as a spoiled newspaper publisher in *The Ghost and Mrs. Muir* (1968–1969)
- Sally Field as *The Flying Nun* and *Gidget*, not to mention *The Girl with Something Extra*
- Goldie Hawn as a body-painted goofball in *Rowan and Martin's Laugh-In* (1968–1972)
- George C. Scott, though he'd appeared in a film or two such as *Anatomy of a Murder*, became known to the public through his series *East Side/West Side* (1963) as a social worker
- Bruce Lee, before he became one of the greatest of all martial-arts stars in film, was the chauffeur Kato in *The Green Hornet* (1966); he inflicted more punishment upon criminals than his trench-coated employer
- Cliff Robertson went on to glory in the movies, but began his career in 1953 as TV's *Rod Brown of the Rocket Rangers*

Robert Shaw, the late actor who starred in *Jaws* and *The Sting*, was the pirate Blackbeard in the 1956 series *The Buccaneer*

Steve McQueen, after a few insignificant films, became a TV hero in *Wanted: Dead or Alive* (1958–1960) as bounty hunter Josh Randall; movie stardom followed when he did *The Great Escape*

Margot Kidder, now a household name thanks to the two Superman films and *The Amityville Horror*, was low woman on the totem in the short-lived James Garner series *Nichols* (1971)

Mark Hamill, none other than the cinema's Luke Skywalker in the *Star Wars* saga, was a co-star on *The Texas Wheelers*, name of Doobie, age sixteen, in 1974

Warren Beatty, one of the top stars by anyone's yardstick, was lowly Milton Armitage on *The Many Loves of Dobie Gillis* (1959–1962)

Long before they became TV superstars, some big names played small supporting roles in the following series:

Marlo Thomas was Stella Barnes in *The Joey Bishop Show* (1961–1964).

Robert Urich, before heading for Las Vegas, was Bob Sanders in *Bob & Carol & Ted & Alice.*

Mary Tyler Moore hadn't co-starred with Dick Van Dyke, let alone created history with her sit com, when only her legs were seen on David Janssen's *Richard Diamond, Private Detective* (1957–1959).

Mike Farrell, who is presently a hit as Capt. B. J. Hunnicut on *M*A*S*H*, where he has resided since 1975, was previously Andy Hays, aide to Mayor Anthony Quinn on the doomed *Man and the City* (1971).

Lee Majors, billed below Barbara Stanwyck, Robert Long, and others on *The Big Valley*, became a star in his own right with *The 6 Million Dollar Man.*

Dan Blocker, who is best known as Hoss Cartwright on *Bonanza*, had actually been featured in another western series previously: he played Tiny Budinger in *Cimarron City* (1958–1959).

Cloris Leachman had appeared in *Lassie*, gaining some fame; before that, however, she had played one Effie Perrine in *Charlie Wild,* a detective show which ran from 1950–1951, a quarter-century before she starred in *Phyllis.*

Adam West, who became a household name as TV's *Batman*, played a crimefighter of a different sort four years earlier: he appeared as Sgt. Steve Nelson on *The Detectives.*

Lightning Strikes Twice

Stars who had hit TV series, whose success was met or surpassed by subsequent series:

Raymond Burr: *Perry Mason* (1957–1965) was a tough act to follow, but Burr had another triumph in *Ironside* (1967–1974)

James Garner: *Maverick* was a legend in its own time, and as Bret Maverick for three of those years Garner was one of the biggest names in TV. Yet, from 1974 through 1980, his *Rockford Files* was no less popular.

Lucille Ball: Though nothing could match the popularity of *I Love Lucy* (1951–1960), the First Lady of TV Comedy actually surpassed the earlier show in terms of years-on-the-air with *The Lucille Ball Show*, known as *The Lucy Show* and *Here's Lucy* later.

Pernell Roberts: The actor quit *Bonanza* after starring in five of its fourteen seasons, dissatisfied with episodic television. However, he returned in *Trapper John, M.D.*, which premiered in 1979 and is still going strong.

Larry Hagman: After making a big impression on the TV public with *I Dream of Jeannie*, Hagman flopped with *The Good Life* (1971), then went supernova as the immortal J. R. Ewing in *Dallas* in 1976.

Barbara Eden: Like Hagman, she was a sensation in *I Dream of Jeannie*. Then, after making TV movies and doing concerts, she returned to weekly TV in 1980 with *Harper Valley P.T.A.*, which was based on her film of the same name and became an instant hit.

Bill Bixby: He *does* have a way with odd companions. Co-starred with an alien in *My Favorite Martian*, he had an even bigger hit playing a part-time monster in *The Incredible Hulk*. There were some other shows in between, such as *The Magician* (1973) and the more successful *Courtship of Eddie's Father*, making Bixby one of TV's most resilient actors.

Ron Howard: He played young Opie Taylor in *The Andy Griffith Show*, then played young Richie Cunningham on *Happy Days*.

Robert Young: All but typecast as Jim Anderson on *Father Knows Best* (1954–1962), he rebounded as *Marcus Welby, M.D.* from 1969–1975.

Mickey Dolenz: As child star Mickey Braddock, he played *Circus Boy* (1956–1957), a show which gained fame in reruns, primarily; from 1966–1967 he was one of *The Monkees*.

Efram Zimbalist, Jr.: As if the hit series *77 Sunset Strip* were not enough, he came back as Inspector Lew Erskine in *The F.B.I.*; remarkably, that's sixteen years of prime-time TV!

Buddy Ebsen: he struck bubblin' crude in *The Beverly Hillbillies* (1962–1976) as Jed Clampett; then came back as a private investigator in *Barnaby Jones* (1973–1979).

What's in a Name?

The real names of some famous TV personalities:

Adam West (*Batman*): Bill Anderson
Eddie Albert (*Switch*): Edward Heimberger
Beatrice Arthur (*Maude*): Bernice Frankel
Robert Blake (*Baretta*): Michael Gubitosi
Diahann Carroll (*Julia*): Carol Diahann Johnson
Angie Dickinson (*Police Woman*): Angeline Brown
James Garner (*Maverick, The Rockford Files*): James Baumgarner
Rock Hudson (*McMillan and Wife*): Roy Scherer, Jr.
Hal Linden (*Barney Miller*): Hal Lipshitz
Ricky Nelson (*The Adventures of Ozzie and Harriet*): Eric Hilliard Nelson
Bob Newhart (*The Bob Newhart Show*): George Newhart
Bernadette Peters (*All's Fair*): Bernadette Lazzara
Telly Savalas (*Kojak*): Aristoteles Savalas
Dinah Shore (*The Dinah Shore Show*): Frances Rose Shore
Suzanne Somers (*Three Company*): Suzanne Mahoney
Marlo Thomas (*That Girl*): Margaret Thomas
Lily Tomlin (*Rowan and Martin's Laugh-In*): Mary Jean Tomlin
Mike Wallace (*60 Minutes*): Myron Wallace
Andy Williams (*The Andy Williams Show*): Howard Williams
Flip Wilson (*The Flip Wilson Show*): Clerow Wilson

Birth dates of some famous TV personalities:

Henry Winkler (*Happy Days*): October 30, 1945
Cindy Williams (*Laverne & Shirley*): August 22, 1948
Mike Wallace (*60Minutes*): May 9, 1918
Robert Wagner (*It Takes a Thief*; *Switch*; *Hart to Hart*): February 10, 1930
Sally Struthers (*All in the Family*): July 28, 1948
Suzanne Somers (*Three's Company*): October 16, 1945
Tom Snyder (*The Tomorrow Show*): May 12, 1936
Jaclyn Smith (*Charlie's Angels*): October 26, 1947
Alan Alda (*M*A*S*H*): January 28, 1936
Ed Asner (*Lou Grant*): November 15, 1929
Lucille Ball (*I Love Lucy*): August 6, 1911
John Belushi (*Saturday Night Live*): January 24, 1948
Carol Burnett (*The Carol Burnett Show*): April 26, 1933
Diahann Carroll (*Julia*): July 17, 1935
David Carradine (*Kung Fu*): December 8, 1936
Johnny Carson (*The Tonight Show Starring Johnny Carson*): October 23, 1925
Dick Cavett (*The Dick Cavett Show*): November 19, 1936
Richard Chamberlain (*Dr. Kildare*): March 31, 1935
Angie Dickinson (*Police Woman*): September 30, 1932
Phil Donahue (*The Phil Donahue Show*): December 21, 1935
Mike Douglas (*The Mike Douglas Show*): August 11, 1925
Mia Farrow (*Peyton Place*): February 9, 1946

Farrah Fawcett (*Charlie's Angels*): February 2, 1947
Sally Field (*Gidget*; *The Flying Nun*): November 6, 1946
Redd Foxx (*Sanford and Son*): December 9, 1922
Valerie Harper (*Rhoda*): August 22, 1940
David Hartman (*Good Morning America*): May 19, 1935
Ron Howard (*Happy Days*): March 1, 1954
Kate Jackson (*Charlie's Angels*): October 29, 1948
Jack Klugman (*Quincy*; *The Odd Couple*): April 27, 1922
Cheryl Ladd (*Charlie's Angels*): April 2, 1950
Cloris Leachman (*Phyllis*): April 30, 1925
Hal Linden (*Barney Miller*): March 20, 1931
Paul Lynde (*The Hollywood Squares*): June 13, 1926
Kristy McNichol (*Family*): September 9, 1962
Lee Majors (*The 6 Million Dollar Man*): April 23, 1940
Mary Tyler Moore (*The Mary Tyler Moore Show*): December 29, 1937
Carroll O'Connor (*All in the Family*): August 2, 1924
Jane Pauley (*The Today Show*): October 31, 1950
John Ritter (*Three's Company*): September 17, 1948

Home-town Folk

The following TV stars may have made it big in Hollywood, but many of them started out in often less-than-glamorous surroundings:

Tony Randall (*The Odd Couple*; *Sidney Shorr*): Tulsa, Oklahoma

Jim Nabors (*Gomer Pyle, U.S.M.C.*): Sylacauga, Alabama

Gilda Radner (*Saturday Night Live*): Detroit, Michigan

Tom Brokaw (*The Today Show*): Webster, South Dakota

David Hartman (*Good Morning America*): Pawtucket, Rhode Island

Ted Knight (*The Mary Tyler Moore Show*): Terryville, Connecticut

Dan Rather (*The CBS Evening News*): Wharton, Texas

Johnny Carson (*The Tonight Show Starring Johnny Carson*): Corning, Iowa

Dick Cavett (*The Dick Cavett Show*): Kearney, Nebraska

Dick Clark (*American Bandstand*): Mt. Vernon, New York

Perry Como (*The Perry Como Show*): Canonsburg, Pennsylvania

John Davidson (*That's Incredible*): Pittsburgh, Pennsylvania

Farrah Fawcett (*Charlie's Angels*): Corpus Christi, Texas

Redd Foxx (*Sanford and Son*): St. Louis, Missouri

Robert Blake (*Baretta*): Nutley, New Jersey

Adam West (*Batman*): Walla Walla, Washington

The following TV series were about the off-screen life of an actor or actress:

The Imogene Coca Show (1954): starring Miss Coca as Betty Crane, a TV comedienne

The Mary Tyler Moore Comedy Hour (1979): short-lived comedy series about the on- and off-tube life of a TV singer-dancer-actress

The Betty White Show (1977): Miss White as Joyce Whitman, the star of the TV series called *Undercover Woman*

The Hero (1966): the story of the off-camera life of western star Sam Garret, who played the tough *Jed Clayton, U.S. Marshal* on TV—but was timid in real life; Garret was played by Richard Mulligan

He & She (1967–1969): Richard Benjamin was cartoonist Dick Hollister, whose comic-strip character Jetman was made into a TV show; co-starred was Jack Cassidy as Oscar North, who played Jetman

Bracken's World (1969): not only the lives of actors and actresses, but the doings in the executive suites of Century Studios

Lorne Green's Favorite TV Shows

The star of *Bonanza* and *Battlestar Galactica* selects these as his personal favorites:

1. *Lou Grant*
2. *The Hill Street Blues*
3. *All in the Family* ("A breakthrough series")
4. *Bonanza*
5. *I Love Lucy* ("When it comes on, I wait and watch it and laugh all over again")
6. *Roots* ("It was a miniseries,, and I *was* in it, but it was still outstanding")
7. *The Waltons*

Some Spin-offs

Series which gave birth to yet other series:

All in the Family: *Maude*; *The Jeffersons*
Maude: *Good Times*
Soap: *Benson*
Alice: *Flo*
Happy Days: Laverne & Shirley
Sanford and Son: *Grady*
The Mary Tyler Moore Show: Lou Grant; Rhoda; Phyllis
Three's Company: *The Ropers*
Barney Miller: *Fish*
*M*A*S*H: Trapper John, M.D.*
The 6 Million Dollar Man: *The Bionic Woman*
The Man from U.N.C.L.E.: *The Girl from U.N.C.L.E.*
Columbo: *Kate Columbo*

First-name Basis

Famous actors who came to TV from the movies or from other series, and played characters with the same first names as their own:

Celeste Holm was Celeste Anders in *Honestly Celeste* (1954).

Mary Tyler Moore was Mary Richards on *The Mary Tyler Moore Show* (1970–1976).

Shirley MacLaine was Shirley Logan on *Shirley's World* (1971).

Doris Day was Doris Martin on *The Doris Day Show* (1968–1972).

Donna Reed was Donna Stone on *The Donna Reed Show* (1958–1965).

Don Rickles was Don Robinson on *The Don Rickles Show* (1972).

Debbie Reynolds was Debbie Thompson on *The Debbie Reynolds Show* (1969).

Phyllis Diller played Phyllis Pruitt on *The Pruitts of Southampton* (1966).

Diana Rigg played Diana Smythe on *Diana* (1973).

Dick Van Dyke was Dick Preston on *The New Dick Van Dyke Show* (1971–1973).

Andy Griffith was Andy Taylor on *The Andy Griffith Show* (1960–1967).

Andy Griffith became Andy Sawyer for *The New Andy Griffith Show* (1971).

Bing Crosby portrayed Bing Collins on *The Bing Crosby Show* (1964).

James Stewart was James Howard on *The Jimmy Stewart Show* (1971).

Lucille Ball was Lucy Carmichael on *The Lucy Show* (1962–1973).

Lucille Ball had previously been Lucy Ricardo on *I Love Lucy* (1951–1960).

Joan Davis starred as Joan Stevens in *I Married Joan* (1952–1954).

Janis Paige was Janis Stewart in *It's Always Jan* (1955).

Robert Cummings played Robert Beanblossom in *My Hero* (1952).

Paul Lynde was Paul Simms on *The Paul Lynde Show* (1972).

Tom Ewell was Tom Potter on *The Tom Ewell Show* (1960).

Bob Newhart played Bob Hartley on *The Bob Newhart Show* (1972–1977).

Bob Crane was Bob Wilcox on *The Bob Crane Show* (1975).

Bob Cummings strikes again, as Bob Collins on *The Bob Cummings Show* (1955–1958).

Robert Urich was Robert Sanders on *Bob & Carol Ted & Alice.*

Ted Knight was Ted Baxter on *The Mary Tyler Moore Show.*

Robert Cummings, cinching the triple crown, played Robert McDonald on *My Living Doll* (1964).

Sally Field was Sally Burton in *The Girl with Something Extra.*

Joey Bishop was Joey Barnes on *The Joey Bishop Show* (1961–1964).

Eve Arden was Eve Hubbard; and Kaye Ballard was Kay Buell; and Roger Carmel as Roger Buell; and Herbert Rudley as Herbert Hubbard; and Jerry Fogel as Jerry Buell in *The Mothers-in-Law* (1967–1968).

Ray Bolger was Ray Wallace on *The Ray Bolger Show* (1953–1954).

Joe Namath was Joe Casey on *The Waverly Wonders* (1978).

First-name Basis (continued)

Gabe Kaplan was Gabe Kotter on *Welcome Back, Kotter* (1975–1979).

Eddie Foy, Jr., was Eddie Walker on *Fair Exchange* (1962).

Danny Thomas was Danny Williams on *Make Room for Daddy* (1953–1964).

Patty Duke was Patty Lane on *The Patty Duke Show* (1963–1965).

Nancy Walker was Nancy Kitteridge on *The Nancy Walker Show* (1976).

Jim Bouton was Jim Barton on *Ball Four* (1976).

Glynis Johns was Glynis Granville on *Glynis* (1963–1964), just as Keith Andes was Keith Granville.

Comedic or dramatic TV series about athletics:

Ball Four (1976): Jim Bouton's book as a series about baseball's Washington Americans
The White Shadow: Ken Howard as a high-school basketball coach
The Bad News Bears: little-league antics
The Bill Cosby Show (1969–1970): Cosby as a phys-ed director in an L.A. school
Where's Huddles: animated series about the football team the Rhinos
The Waverly Wonders: Joe Namath as a high-school basketball coach

The highest-rated theatrical motion pictures ever shown on prime-time TV (note: applies to first-run features only):

1. *Gone With the Wind* (Part One)
2. *Gone With the Wind* (Part Two)
3. *Airport*
4. *Love Story*
5. *The Godfather* (Part Two of two parts; not the film of the same name)
6. *Jaws*
7. *The Poseidon Adventure*
8. *True Grit*
9. *The Birds*
10. *Patton*
11. *Bridge on the River Kwai*
12. *Jeremiah Johnson*
13. *Ben-Hur*
14. *Rocky*
15. *The Godfather* (Part One)
16. *The Wizard of Oz* (annually garnering roughly this position in the ratings)
17. *Planets of the Apes*
18. *Born Free*
19. *The Sound of Music*
20. *Bonnie and Clyde*
21. *The Ten Commandments* (like *The Wizard of Oz,* winning a yearly spot on the list, this being the highest mark it ever achieved)
22. *The Longest Yard*
23. *Beneath the Planet of the Apes*
24. *Cat on a Hot Tin Roof*
25. *Skyjacked*

26. *The Apple Dumpling Gang*
27. *Butch Cassidy and the Sundance Kid*
28. *The Sting*
29. *Smokey and the Bandit*
30. *Oh, God!*
31. *Airport 1975*
32. *The Great Escape* (Part Two)
33. *McLintock*
34. *The Ballad of Josie*
35. *The Great Escape* (Part One)
36. *Goldfinger*
37. *The Robe*
38. *Three Days of the Condor*
39. *The Graduate*
40. *The Dirty Dozen*
41. *Earthquake* (Part Two) (Part One, without the disaster scenes, is #69)
42. *The War Wagon*
43. *Lilies of the Field*
44. *Your Cheatin' Heart*
45. *Gidget Goes Hawaiian*
46. *Five Branded Women*
47. *Hooper*
48. *PT 109*
49. *Escape from the Planet of the Apes*
50. *Roustabout*

The top-rated made-for-television movies in history:

1. *Helter Skelter* (Part Two)
2. *Little Ladies of the Night*
3. *Helter Skelter* (Part One)
4. *The Waltons' Thanksgiving Story*
5. *The Night Stalker*
6. *A Case of Rape*
7. *The Dallas Cowboys Cheerleaders*
8. *Brian's Song*
9. *Women in Chains*
10. *Jesus of Nazareth* (Part One)
11. *Heidi*
12. *My Sweet Charlie*
13. *The Feminist and the Fuzz*
14. *Something for Joey*
15. *Dawn: Portrait of a Teenage Runaway*
16. *The Amazing Howard Hughes* (Part Two)
17. *Sarah T.—Portrait of a Teenage Alcoholic*
18. *Call Her Mom*
19. *Death of Innocence*
20. *The Autobiography of Miss Jane Pitman*
21. *Charlie's Angels*
22. *Rescue from Gilligan's Island*
23. *Tribes*
24. *Yuma*
25. *Mr. & Mrs. Bo-Jo Jones*
26. *Melvin Purvis, G-Man*
27. *Mrs. Sundance*
28. *The Waltons' Easter Story*
29. *Maybe I'll come Home in the Spring*
30. *Jesus of Nazareth* (Part Two)
31. *Alias Smith and Jones*

32. *Raid on Entebbe*
33. *The Homecoming*
34. *Sibyl*
35. *The Incredible Journey of Dr. Meg Laurel*
36. *Gidget Gets Married*
37. *The Jericho Mile*
38. *The Runaways*
39. *Dr. Cook's Garden*
40. *Flying High*
41. *The Last Child*
42. *Battlestar Galactica*
43. *SST—Death Flight*
44. *The Girl Most Likely To*
45. *In Search of America*
46. *Cry Rape!*
47. *Wild Women*
48. *Doomsday Flight*
49. *The Longest Hundred Miles*
50. *The Red Pony*

Virtually since its inception, television has been a medium of competition—not just athletic competition, or the tilts between dramatic antagonists, but competition for the attention of audiences nationwide. Thus, almost hand in hand with the coming of sponsored TV came ratings for TV programs: analyses, based upon representative samplings, of how many people are watching a given show at a given time. The leader of the ratings gathering has always been the A. C. Nielsen Company. However, whereas it once took days to assimilate and report on the data, it is now a matter of hours; shows which were in ratings trouble were rarely canceled before the full September-to-September season had been carefully rated, changes made, the changes rated, and the show finally judged. Today, because of the massive advertising revenue derived by TV, shows which do not perform may not last through the morning after their debut. A perfect example was *Turn-On*, which premiered on February 5, 1969, and died the very next morning. Here, as a point of curiosity, are the ratings for the first full-fledged TV season, which ran from October of 1950 through the spring of 1951:

1. *Texaco Star Theatre (The Milton Berle Show)*: 61.6
2. *Fireside Theatre*: 52.6
3. *Philco TV Playhouse*: 45.3
4. *Your Show of Shows*: 42.6
5. *The Colgate Comedy Hour*: 42
6. *Gillette Cavalcade of Sports*: 41.3
7. *The Lone Ranger*: 41.2

TV's Top Ten (continued)

8. *Arthur Godfrey's Talent Scouts*: 40.6
9. *Hopalong Cassidy*: 39.9
10. *Mama*: 39.7

The numbers cited beside each show represents, of those homes with TVs, the percentage tuned in to that program. Pressing on through the succession on TV seasons, we find the following series to have been the winners of each annual tally:

1951–1952

1. *Arthur Godfrey's Talent Scouts*
2. *Texaco Star Theatre*
3. *I Love Lucy*
4. *The Red Skelton Show*
5. *The Colgate Comedy Hour*
6. *Arthur Godfrey and His Friends*
7. *Fireside Theatre*
8. *Your Show of Shows*
9. *The Jack Benny Show*
10. *You Bet Your Life*

1952–1953

1. *I Love Lucy*
2. *Arthur Godfrey's Talent Scouts*
3. *Arthur Godfrey and His Friends*
4. *Dragnet*
5. *Texaco Star Theatre*
6. *The Buick Circus Hour*
7. *The Colgate Comedy Hour*
8. *Gangbusters*
9. *You Bet Your Life*
10. *Fireside Theatre*

1953–1954

1. *I Love Lucy*
2. *Dragnet*
3. *Arthur Godfrey's Talent Scouts*
4. *You Bet Your Life*
5. *The Chevy Show*
6. *The Milton Berle Show*
7. *Arthur Godfrey and His Friends*
8. *The Ford Show*
9. *The Jackie Gleason Show*
10. *Fireside Theatre*

TV's Top Ten (continued)

1954–1955

1. *I Love Lucy*
2. *The Jackie Gleason Show*
3. *Dragnet*
4. *You Bet Your Life*
5. *The Toast of the Town* (Ed Sullivan)
6. *Disneyland*
7. *The Chevy Show*
8. *The Jack Benny Show*
9. *The Martha Raye Show*
10. *The George Gobel Show*

1955–1956

1. *The $64,000 Question*
2. *I Love Lucy*
3. *The Ed Sullivan Show Show*
4. *Disneyland*
5. *The Jack Benny Show Show*
6. *December Bride*
7. *You Bet Your Life*
8. *Dragnet*
9. *The Millionaire*
10. *I've Got a Secret*

1956–1957

1. *I Love Lucy*
2. *The Ed Sullivan Show*
3. *General Electric Theatre*
4. *The $64,000 Question*
5. *December Bride*
6. *Alfred Hitchcock Presents*
7. *I've Got a Secret*
8. *Gunsmoke*
9. *The Perry Como Show*
10. *The Jack Benny Show*

1957–1958

1. *Gunsmoke*
2. *The Danny Thomas Show*
3. *Tales of Wells Fargo*
4. *Have Gun Will Travel*
5. *I've Got a Secret*
6. *The Life and Legend of Wyatt Earp*
7. *General Electric Theatre*
8. *The Restless Gun*
9. *December Bride*
10. *You Bet Your Life*

1958–1959

1. *Gunsmoke*
2. *Wagon Train*
3. *Have Gun Will Travel*

TV's Top Ten (continued)

4. *The Rifleman*
5. *The Danny Thomas Show*
6. *Maverick*
7. *Tales of Wells Fargo*
8. *The Real McCoys*
9. *I've Got a Secret*
10. *The Life and Legend of Wyatt Earp*

1959–1960

1. *Gunsmoke*
2. *Wagon Train*
3. *Have Gun Will Travel*
4. *The Danny Thomas Show*
5. *The Red Skelton Show*
6. *Father Knows Best*
7. *77 Sunset Strip*
8. *The Price Is Right*
9. *Wanted: Dead or Alive*
10. *Perry Mason*

1960–1961

1. *Gunsmoke*
2. *Wagon Train*
3. *Have Gun Will Travel*
4. *The Andy Griffith Show*
5. *The Real McCoys*
6. *Rawhide*
7. *Candid Camera*
8. *The Untouchables*
9. *The Price Is Right*
10. *The Jack Benny Show*

1961–1962

1. *Wagon Train*
2. *Bonanza*
3. *Gunsmoke*
4. *Hazel*
5. *Perry Mason*
6. *The Red Skelton Show*
7. *The Andy Griffith Show*
8. *The Danny Thomas Show*
9. *Dr. Kildare*
10. *Candid Camera*

1962–1963

1. *The Beverly Hillbillies*
2. *The Red Skelton Show*
3. *Candid Camera*
4. *Bonanza*
5. *The Lucy Show*
6. *The Andy Griffith Show*

7. *The Danny Thomas Show*
8. *Ben Casey*
9. *The Dick Van Dyke Show*
10. *Gunsmoke*

1963–1964

1. *The Beverly Hillbillies*
2. *Bonanza*
3. *The Dick Van Dyke Show*
4. *Petticoat Junction*
5. *The Andy Griffith Show*
6. *The Lucy Show*
7. *Candid Camera*
8. *The Ed Sullivan Show*
9. *The Danny Thomas Show*
10. *My Favorite Martian*

1964–1965

1. *Bonanza*
2. *Bewitched*
3. *Gomer Pyle, U.S.M.C.*
4. *The Andy Griffith Show*
5. *The Fugitive*
6. *The Red Skelton Hour*
7. *The Dick Van Dyke Show*
8. *The Lucy Show*
9. *Peyton Place*
10. *Combat*

1965–1966

1. *Bonanza*
2. *Gomer Pyle, U.S.M.C.*
3. *The Lucy Show*
4. *The Red Skelton Hour*
5. *Batman* (the Thursday-night segment, second of two)
6. *The Andy Griffith Show*
7. *The Beverly Hillbillies*
8. *Bewitched*
9. *Hogan's Heroes*
10. *Batman* (the Wednesday-night segment)

1966–1967

1. *Bonanza*
2. *The Red Skelton Hour*
3. *The Andy Griffith Show*

4. *The Lucy Show*
5. *The Jackie Gleason Show*
6. *Green Acres*
7. *Daktari*
8. *The Beverly Hillbillies*
9. *Bewitched*
10. *The Lawrence Welk Show*

1967–1968

1. *The Andy Griffith Show*
2. *The Lucy Show*
3. *Gomer Pyle, U.S.M.C.*
4. *Gunsmoke*
5. *Bonanza*
6. *Family Affair*
7. *The Red Skelton Show*
8. *The Dean Martin Show*
9. *The Jackie Gleason Show*
10. *Saturday Night at the Movies*

1968–1969

1. *Rowan & Martin's Laugh-In*
2. *Gomer Pyle, U.S.M.C.*
3. *Bonanza*
4. *Mayberry R.F.D.*
5. *Family Affair*
6. *Gunsmoke*
7. *Julia*
8. *The Dean Martin Show*
9. *Here's Lucy: (The Lucy Show)*
10. *The Beverly Hillbillies*

1969–1970

1. *Rowan & Martin's Laugh-In*
2. *Gunsmoke*
3. *Bonanza*
4. *Mayberry R.F.D.*
5. *Family Affair*
6. *Here's Lucy*
7. *The Red Skelton Hour*
8. *Marcus Welby, M.D.*
9. *Walt Disney's Wonderful World of Color*
10. *The Doris Day Show*

1970–1971

1. *Marcus Welby, M.D.*
2. *The Flip Wilson Show*

3. *Here's Lucy*
4. *Ironside*
5. *Gunsmoke*
6. *ABC Movie of the Week*
7. *Hawaii Five-O*
8. *Medical Center*
9. *Bonanza*
10. *The F.B.I.*

1971–1972

1. *All in the Family*
2. *The Flip Wilson Show*
3. *Marcus Welby, M.D.*
4. *Gunsmoke*
5. *ABC Movie of the Week*
6. *Sanford and Son*
7. *Mannix*
8. *Funny Face*
9. *Adam 12*
10. *The Mary Tyler Moore Show*

1972–1973

1. *All in the Family*
2. *Sanford and Son*
3. *Hawaii Five-O*
4. *Maude*
5. *NBC Sunday Mystery Movie* (featuring *McMillan and Wife, McCloud,* and *Columbo)*
6. *Bridget Loves Bernie*
7. *The Mary Tyler Moore Show*
8. *Gunsmoke*
9. *The Wonderful World of Disney*
10. *Ironside*

1973–1974

1. *All in the Family*
2. *The Waltons*
3. *Sanford and Son*
4. *M*A*S*H*
5. *Hawaii Five-O*
6. *Maude*
7. *Kojak*
8. *The Sonny and Cher Comedy Hour*
9. *Cannon*
10. *The Mary Tyler Moore Show*

1974–1975

1. *All in the Family*
2. *Sanford and Son*
3. *Chico and the Man*
4. *The Jeffersons*
5. *M*A*S*H*
6. *Good Times*
7. *Rhoda*

TV's Top Ten (continued)

8. *The Waltons*
9. *Maude*
10. *Hawaii Five-O*

1975–1976

1. *All in the Family*
2. *Lavern & Shirley*
3. *Maude*
4. *The Bionic Woman*
5. *Phyllis*
6. *Sanford and Son*
7. *Rhoda*
8. *The 6 Million Dollar Man*
9. *ABC Monday Night Movie*
10. *Happy Days*

1976–1977

1. *Happy Days*
2. *Laverne & Shirley*
3. *ABC Monday Night Movie*
4. *M*A*S*H*
5. *Charlie's Angels*
6. *The Big Event*
7. *The 6 Million Dollar Man*
8. *Baretta*
9. *ABC Sunday Night Movie*
10. *One Day at a Time*

1977–1978

1. *Laverne & Shirley*
2. *Happy Days*
3. *Three's Company*
4. *60 Minutes*
5. *All in the Family*
6. *Charlie's Angels*
7. *Little House on the Prairie*
8. *M*A*S*H*
9. *Alice*
10. *One Day at a Time*

1978–1979

1. *Three's Company*
2. *Laverne & Shirley*
3. *Mork and Mindy*
4. *Happy Days*
5. *Angie*
6. *60 Minutes*
7. *M*A*S*H*
8. *The Ropers*
9. *Charlie's Angels*
10. *Taxi*

TV series whose musical themes became hit records:

All in the Family
Baretta
Batman
Ben Casey
The Beverly Hillbillies
Bonanza
Charlie's Angels
Dragnet
The Greatest American Hero
The Green Hornet
Happy Days
Have Gun Will Travel
Hawaii Five-O
Here Come the Brides
I Love Lucy (disco version)
Laverne & Shirley
The Men
Mission: Impossible
Mr. Lucky
My Three Sons
Peter Gunn
The Rockford Files
Route 66
S.W.A.T.
Secret Agent
Welcome Back, Kotter
Zorro

The average cost of some favorite TV shows, per episode:

Archie Bunker's Place: $275,000
Barney Miller: $250,000
Battlestar Galactica: $750,000 (over half of it in special effects)
Buck Rogers in the 25th Century: $800,000 (half in effects work)
Charlie's Angels: $500,000
Dallas: $500,000 (much of it in salaries)
Fantasy Island: $500,000
Happy Days: $300,000
The Incredible Hulk: $575,000
Magnum, P.I.: $625,000
*M*A*S*H*: $250,000
Mork & Mindy: $250,000
6 Million Dollar Man: $500,000
Three's Company: $210,000 (high salaries)
The Waltons: $450,000

More than Whole

Movies made for theatrical release, which have had scenes *added* for television showings:

Airport 1977: Expanded with cut footage to stretch the boredom.

King Kong: Became two rather than one night of utter trash.

Two-Minute Warning: The story of a mad sniper had new scenes filmed to become an art heist!

The Godfather and *The Godfather Part Two*: merged and expanded with excised scenes.

The Hindenburg: Only five minutes of film, left on the cutting-room floor, were slipped back in to this underrated historical epic.

Earthquake: A fairly substantial subplot was deleted from the theatrical film in 1974. It involved an airplane headed for a landing in Los Angeles, trying to touch down just as the city goes to pieces. The aircraft manages to rev up and leave the runway, which is breaking up beneath it. The scenes were cut originally so as not to compete with the same studio's *Airport 1975,* released weeks earlier. Other, slow scenes involving Marjoe Gortner and Victoria Principal were also retrieved from the cutting room.

Star Trek: The Motion Picture: Due to an encroaching release date, director Robert Wise and his special-effects team were literally unable to complete their film, leaving several special effects and their pertinent live-action scenes in the can. Several of these have been restored.

Lawrence of Arabia and *Ben-Hur*: Both superepics were edited for theatrical rerelease. When shown on TV, the snipped sequences were restored.

Buck Rogers in the 25th Century: You'll have to pay attention on this one. The film was originally made for television, but the producers decided to release it first theatrically. Wise move—it made tens of millions of dollars. In translating the TV film to a theatrical feature, some additional, spectacular action scenes were shot, along with some sex and profanity and violence. Bringing the movie *back* to TV, the added matter was snipped out—and *new* footage put in, since the feature was now the first episode of a new series. The new scenes introduced Buck (and the viewer) to his twenty-fifth century apartment, and so on.

Pop Lingo

Words or phrases from TV shows which, for a time, leaped from the lips of every other person one met:

"Sorry about that, Chief!" from *Get Smart*
"Dy-no-*mite*!" from *Good Times*
"Shazam!" from *Gomer Pyle, U.S.M.C.*
"Ayyyyyyy . . ." from *Happy Days*
"Would you believe . . . ?" also from *Get Smart*
"Holy *(fill in the blank)*" from *Batman*
"Up your nose with a rubber hose" from *Welcome Back, Kotter*
"Nanu, nanu" from *Mork and Mindy*
"Who loves ya, baby?" from *Kojak*
"*V*errrry interesting" from *Rowan & Martin's Laugh-In*
"Sock-it-to-me" from *Rowan & Martin's Laugh-In*
"Here come da judge" from, one more time, *Rowan & Martin's Laugh-In*
"Smile! You're on *Candid Camera*!" from *Candid Camera*
"How (hot, short, tall, fast, etc.) *was* it?" from *The Tonight Show Starring Johnny Carson*

Characters who have been killed during the run of a series so the actors themselves could move on:

Edith Bunker (Jean Stapleton) on *Archie Bunker's Place*
Brigadier General Frank Savage (Robert Lansing) on *Twelve O'Clock High*
Lieutenant Colonel Henry Blake (McLean Stevenson) on *M*A*S*H*
Captain Apollo (Richard Hatch) on *Galactica: 1980*

. . . and several who died during the run of a series:

Joan Bradford (Diana Hyland) on *Eight Is Enough*
Detective Yemana (Jack Soo) on *Barney Miller*
Grandpa Walton (Will Geer) on *The Waltons*
Hoss Cartwright (Dan Blocker) on *Bonanza*
Julie Erskine (Barbara Colby) on *Phyllis*
George Wilson (Joseph Kearns) on *Dennis the Menace*
Major Seth Adams (Ward Bond) on *Wagon Train*
Chico Rodriguez (Freddie Prinze) on *Chico and the Man*

Coming of Age

A sampling of red-letter dates in the history of television:

TV patent first applied for in 1924.

TV begins "officially" in 1926 as NBC broadcasts a grand ball from the Waldorf-Astoria Hotel in New York.

NBC broadcasts the opening ceremonies of the New York World's Fair in May 1939.

Color TV is unveiled in September 1940, though not yet commercially available.

The first "network" is set up between Philadelphia and Washington by Philco in April 1945 as an alternative to regional programming.

The first full broadcast of an opera, *Otello*, is aired on ABC in December 1948.

The first telecast of a presidential inauguration, that of Harry Truman, in January 1949.

September 1950: the first World Series sportscast.

In September of 1951, the first nationwide simulcasts are established.

TV Guide magazine appears, metamorphosed from *TV Digest* of Philadelphia, in April 1953, and becomes the most popular periodical in the United States.

President Eisenhower holds the first televised news conference in January 1954.

The first Kennedy-Nixon debate in October 1960.

Kennedy puts a program into motion to use satellites as communications and broadcast media in July 1961.

No more cables, no more delayed and fuzzy pictures: the satellite Telstar fulfills Kennedy's dream, making possible instant worldwide broadcasting in July 1962.

Astronaut L. Gordon Cooper broadcasts the first live pictures from space, with a camera perched inside his Mercury spacecraft.

Coverage of the assassination of President Kennedy in November 1963 simultaneously matures the impact of television as a news medium.

The first lunar broadcast, by camera person Neil A. Armstrong, on July 20, 1969.

Cigarette advertising banned in January 1971.

Name That Tune

A change-of-pace list: lines from the theme songs of TV series. As an added bit of amusement, we've listed the titles below; try to guess them without peeking!

"There's miracles a-start, but they always come apart . . ."
"It's about two astronauts, it's about their fate . . ."
"There's a holdup in the Bronx, Brooklyn's broken out in fights . . ."
"Look! It's the man who flies around like an eagle!"
"For he lived what he had known, and he reaped what he had sown—and the world will not forget . . ."
"You're doomed to wander, on beyond this land so lonely . . ."
"Look at what's happened to me. I still can't believe it myself . . ."
"Here we come, walkin' down the street, get the funniest looks from everyone we meet . . ."
"Out of the night when the full moon is bright . . ."
"Come and listen to a story 'bout a man named Jed, a poor mountaineer barely kept his family fed . . ."
"Welcome back, your dreams were your ticket out . . ."
"They've given you a number and they've taken 'way your name."
"Who can take a rainy day, and suddenly make it all seem worthwhile?"

The Smothers Brothers Show
It's About Time (1966)
Car 54, Where Are You? (1961–1962)
Captain Nice (1967)
The Legend of Jesse James

Name That Tune (continued)

A Man Called Shenandoah (1965)
The Greatest American Hero (1980–present)
The Monkees
Zorro
The Beverly Hillbillies
Welcome Back, Kotter
Secret Agent (1965)
The Mary Tyler Moore Show

Didja Know . . . ?

An assortment of facts and observations about TV programs; didja know, for example . . .

. . . that after making a few films in which he was barely noticed, and prior to starring as *The Saint*, Roger Moore appeared in two U.S. TV series: *The Alaskans* (1959) and *Maverick* (for one season, 1960)?

. . . that Sam the Bartender on *Gunsmoke* (he appeared from 1962–1974) was the late actor Glenn Strange, whose only other claim to fame was having starred as the Frankenstein monster in the waning years of that popular series?

. . . Sally Struthers, who is best known as Gloria on *All in the Family*, was for a single season a regular on *The Smothers Brothers Comedy Hour*?

. . . *The Green Hornet*, who lasted only a single season (1966) on TV, is in his secret identity Britt Reid . . . a descendant of *The Long Ranger*, alias John Reid?

. . . Rod Serling, who won a fistful of Emmy awards as a writer and host of *The Twilight Zone*, created two instant-flop series before he returned in the successful *Night Gallery*? The failures: a magnificent western show starring Lloyd Bridges and called *The Loner* (1965), and a silly *Lord of the Flies* show with grown-ups entitled *The New People*, about a planeload of passengers who crash on a remote isle and form a microcosm of society thereupon, that loser in 1969.

. . . numerous actors who created classic roles for TV did not get to play those parts in the film version: for example, Jack Palance in *Requiem for a Heavy-*

weight (enter Anthony Quinn); Rod Steiger for *Marty* (an Oscar for Ernest Borgnine); Cliff Robertson for *Days of Wine and Roses* (acclaim for Jack Lemmon); and many others.

. . . that there was actually a regularly scheduled series dramatizing the lives of postal carriers? Not a sit com, mind you, but *drama*? The show was called, forthrightly, *The Mail Story*, and ABC had it for two months in the fall of 1954.

. . . numerous American series have been based on hit British shows, for example *All in the Family* (*Till Death Do Us Part*), *Lotsa Luck* (*On the Busses*), *Three's Company* (*Man About the House*), and many more.

. . . until the middle of 1981, Milton Berle was receiving $200,000 per year from NBC, even though his show had long gone off the air; he signed the thirty-year contract at the height of his popularity, which appeared as though it would never wane.

A Hit by Any Other Name

Often, to avoid confusion in the public's mind, a network program which goes into syndication—that is, reruns sold to local stations—undergoes a title change. Here are a few:

Wagon Train became *Major Adams, Trailmaster*
Fury became *Brave Stallion*
The Andy Griffith Show became *Andy of Mayberry*
Dragnet became *Badge 714*
Bonanza became *Ponderosa* (both on network TV; the latter being reruns)
Richard Diamond, Private Detective became *Call Mr. D*
Gangbusters became *Captured*
Mark Saber became *Detective's Diary*
Treasury Men in Action became *Federal Men*
Gunsmoke became *Marshal Dillon* (both on network TV again, the latter reruns)
Big Town became *Heart of the City*
Have Gun Will Travel became *Paladin*
The Millionaire became *If You Had a Million*
Lassie became *Jeff's Collie*
The Bob Cummings Show became *Love That Bob*
The Real McCoys became, simply, *The McCoys*
The Gale Storm Show became *Oh, Susanna*
Alcoa Presents became *One Step Beyond*
The Rockford Files became *Jim Rockford, Private Eye*
The Phil Silvers Show became *Sgt. Bilko*

Astound friends and family alike with knowledge of things at once obscure and familiar:

- The name of *Sky King's* airplane was *Songbird.*
- The civilian identity of *Batman,* Bruce Wayne, derives from Scotland's King Robert the Bruce, and from American revolutionary war hero "Mad" Anthony Wayne.
- The Osmond Brothers once starred as the Kissel Brothers on a short-lived western series entitled *The Travels of Jamie McPheeters* (1963).
- The panelists on the first season of *To Tell the Truth* were Hy Gardner, Hildy Parks, Polly Bergen, and the perennial Kitty Carlisle.
- On *That Girl,* Ted Bessell's character Don Hollinger worked for *Newsview* magazine.
- Speaking of magazines, on *The Name of the Game* (1968–1970), Robert Stack's Dan Farrell was an editor for *Crime* magazine.
- Merv Griffin's first and biggest hit record was "I've Got a Lovely Bunch of Coconuts."
- Raymond Burr's father was a hardware salesperson in Canada.
- Johnny Carson's middle name is William.
- Desi Arnaz, Jr., was featured on the first cover of *TV Guide.*
- The working title for *All in the Family* was *Those Were the Days.*
- The original choice for Capt. Kirk on *Star Trek* was film star Jeffrey Hunter; he played the role in the show's first pilot. When that failed to sell, a second pilot was made with William Shatner. Footage from

the Hunter pilot was incorporated into a two-part show when the series finally made it onto the air.

- TV is not the only medium which has spin-offs. Radio's *Fibber McGee and Molly* gave birth to *Beulah*, both of which later became TV series in the early 1950s.
- The characterization of the inept Maxwell Smart of *Get Smart* was actually developed by actor Don Adams on *The Bill Dana Show* (1963–1965) in the person of hotel detective Byron Glick.
- Though TV has its superstars, there are many toilers in the vineyard who have been around a *long* time. For instance, Dick Van Patten, who has struck it big with *Eight Is Enough*, has been doing TV for over thirty years; his series include, *Mama* (1949), *The New Dick Van Dyke Show*, *The Partners*, and Mel Brooks' *When Things Were Rotten*.

Holy Malfeasance!

One of the greatest phenomena of TV in the 1960s was the popularity of the *Batman* prime-time series. It aired from 1966–1968, and was an "in" show not only among viewers, but among actors as well. *Everyone* wanted to play one of the program's colorful villains. Here are the few who succeeded:

Frank Gorshin (the Riddler)
Burgess Meredith (the Penguin)
Cesar Romero (the Joker)
George Sanders (Mr. Freeze)
Ann Baxter (Zelda)
David Wayne (the Mad Hatter)
Malachi Throne (False Face)
Julie Newmar (the Catwoman)
Victor Buono (King Tut)
Roddy McDowall (the Bookworm)
Art Carney (the Archer)
Van Johnson (the Minstrel)
Shelley Winters (Ma Parker)
Walter Slezak (the Clock King)
Vincent Price (Egghead)
Liberace (Chandell)
Otto Preminger (Mr. Freeze)
Carolyn Jones (Marsha)
Maurice Evans (the Puzzler)
Michael Rennie (Sandman)
John Astin (the Riddler)
Roger C. Carmel (Colonel Gumm)
Tallulah Bankhead (the Black Widow)
Eli Wallach (Mr. Freeze)
Milton Berle (Louie the Lilac)
Joan Collins (Siren)

Rudy Vallee (Lord Phogg)
Eartha Kitt (Catwoman)
Barbara Rush (Nora Clavicle)
Ida Lupino (Dr. Cassandra)
Cliff Robertson (Shame)
Zsa Zsa Gabor (Minerva)

Big Fizzle

TV stars who tried to go from the small screen to motion pictures and flopped:

Henry Winkler, immortalized on *Happy Days*, died in *Heroes* and *The One and Only*.

William Shatner, deified on *Star Trek*, fell to earth with films like *Kingdom of the Spiders*.

Farrah Fawcett, *the* sex bomb of the 1970s, tried to expand from *Charlie's Angels* in *Somebody Killed Her Husband*, *Sunburn*, and *Saturn III*. All were megaflops.

John Ritter went from *Three's Company* to *Hero at Large* on the silver screen—then returned to TV. The film was underrated, but failed nonetheless.

Lorne Greene will always be Ben Cartwright, despite *Earthquake*, *The Buccaneer*, and others.

Lee Majors, TV's *6 Million Dollar Man*, fared worse than his ex-wife Farrah, flopping in *Steel*, *The Norsemen*, and *The Last Chase*. He, too, has gone back to TV.

Robert Blake, who did so well on *Baretta*, had been an unsuccessful movie star before (*Electra Glide in Blue*) and became one again (*Coast to Coast*)—through no fault of his own, incidentally; he's good in both.

David Hartman, after trying TV and not succeeding very well in *Lucas Tanner* and *The Virginian*, and moderately well as a supporting player in *The New Doctors*, gave movies a try—and helped Walt Disney Productions to one of their few failures with *Island at the Top of the World*. He then single-handedly gave ABC a morning colossus with *Good Morning America.*

David Janssen could do no wrong on the home tube—but in films like *The Green Berets* and *Two-Minute Warning* he was an utter washout.

Chuck Connors, who started by playing heavies in films like *Designing Woman,* came to TV in *The Rifleman,* followed by *Branded* and *Cowboy in Africa.* Despite having made co-starring appearances in films like *Soylent Green* and *Captain Nemo and the Underwater City,* he has been unable to overcome his TV image.

Ron Ely, who was TV's *Tarzan* and host of the game show *Face the Music,* is an actor who, unlike many others, *has* big-screen charisma but has been saddled with losing vehicles. His screen presence in the disastrous *Doc Savage,* a pre-Superman superhero film made in 1975, is nothing short of magnetic.

Adam West, like Ely, *has* what it takes for the movie screen, but has been saddled with the *Batman* image. He has made numerous foreign films, and recently starred in *The Happy Hooker Goes to Hollywood.* He has, of late, done mostly guest spots on programs like *Fantasy Island* as well as many pilots. He was, along with Roger Moore, considered as a replacement for Sean Connery in the James Bond films. Like Ron Ely, West *will* one day soon make it to the big screen in a big way.

It is puzzling to note that even in *good* films, like *Hero at Large,* TV stars are unable to pull in an audience . . . puzzling in that the *weekly* audience of any TV show is usually greater than the top-grossing film of the *year*! Conversely, it is axiomatic in Hollywood that audiences won't pay to see anyone in a theater they can see for free in their home. The reverse is also true: the biggest theatrical stars, as we've noted in another list, fail to draw a TV crowd because while five million movie fans can make a successful film, that's the *worst* kind of television rating.

Mad About TV

Mad magazine, for nearly thirty years one of the nation's top satire publications, has spoofed every aspect of society—including television. Here are a few of the TV parodies they have published over the years:

Star Blecch: the adventures of the starship *Booby-Prize*
Genteel Ben: also known as Trouble is a-bruin'
How-Are-Ya Five-O?: self-proclaimed as aloha-ha-ha
Bananaz: which they dubbed "the four horsemen of the preposterous"
Mission: Ridiculous: complete with a self-destructing bowling-ball tape recorder
The Six Million Dollars, Man!: and his battle with the Ten Million Ruble Woman
Hokum's Heroes: which features a look at an even *more* tasteless show, *Hochman's Heroes*
Gall in the Family Fare: subtitled *Little Bigot Man*
Reality Street: ("Crummy day . . . smoggy sky's charcoal gray. . . .")
Bats-Man: wherein Robin turns on his guardian
Cattlecar Galaxica: better than the series because it's *intentionally* funny
Too Gross for Comfort: kinder than this show deserves

Heard but not Seen

Some stars find they have time on their hands between seasons or could use a few extra dollars; or some did the work before they became famous. Either way, a number of noted TV actors have been the voices of cartoon characters seen on Saturday-morning animated shows. Among them:

Don Adams was *Tennessee Tuxedo* in 1963, before he did *Get Smart*; Larry Storch, later of *F-Troop*, provided the voice for Phineas J. Whoopee on that show.

Adam West, the live-action *Batman*, and Burt Ward, the nonanimated Robin, provided the voices for their cartoon counterparts.

William Shatner, Leonard Nimoy, DeForest Kelley, and the other members of *Star Trek* TV show put words in the mouths of their animated kin.

Ted Knight, just before stardom struck on *The Mary Tyler Moore Show*, did the narration for *Super-Friends.*

Ross Martin, of *The Wild, Wild West*, lent his wonderfully disguisable voice to *Sealab 2020* as Dr. Paul Williams.

Richard Long repeated his role from *Nanny and the Professor*, and Juliet Mills hers on *The Saturday Superstar Movie.*

Dom DeLuise, still largely unknown, played Mr. Evictus on *Roman Holidays* in the early 1970s.

William Conrad, none other than *Cannon*, was the narrator of *Rocky and His Friends.*

Paul Lynde, in his pre-*Holywood Square* days, was Sylvester Sneekly in *The Perils of Penelope Pitstop.*

Sally Struthers, on the eve of her *All in the Family*

fame, was Pebbles Flintstone on *Pebbles and Bamm Bamm.*

The Osmond Brothers were themselves on *The Osmonds.*

Bob Denver, Alan Hale, and company did the honors for *The New Adventures of Gilligan.*

Jonathan Harris, Dr. Smith from *Lost in Space*, was another kind of spacefarer, taking over the part created by Ray Walston for the cartoon *My Favorite Martians.*

Mark Hamill, later of *Star Wars*, played Corry in *Jeannie*, a cartoon version of *I Dream of Jeannie.*

The Jackson Five played themselves on *The Jackson Five.*

Muhammad Ali played *himself* on *I'm the Greatest.*

Mickey Dolenz, through with *The Monkees*, played Skip on *The Funky Phantom.*

Kevin Tighe and Randolph Mantooth both played their live-action characters on *Emergency Plus Four.*

Maureen McCormick, Barry Williams, and siblings all played *The Brady Kids* based on *The Brady Bunch.*

If an idea's weak, the best acting in the world can't save it. Here are some of the nuttier plots which have served as the basis for made-for-TV movies:

The Man with the Power (1977): A teacher learns that his father was a creature from another planet, one who endowed him with extraordinary abilities. The *Superman* motif wasn't bad in itself, until the alien spawn became an agent for the government.

A Cold Night's Death (1973): Robert Culp as a scientist in the Arctic, unaware that he's a pawn in a game being played by superintelligent monkeys.

The Love War (1970): Argon and Zinan are planets at war with each other. Instead of slugging it out on their home turf, the aliens use earth as their arena, adopting human form so as to blend in. When an Argonian falls in love with a Zinanian, this absurd *Romeo and Juliet* becomes laughable.

Poor Devil (1972): Sammy Davis, Jr., is a bumbling devil sent to earth to snare the soul of Jack Klugman. Slapstick and deviltry just don't mix.

Satan's School for Girls (1973): A cross between *The Exorcist* and *The Pure Hell of St. Trinian's*, as the devil goes after a group of co-eds.

The Last Dinosaur (1977): Richard Boone discovers an island inhabited by dinosaurs and, rather than study them, grabs an elephant gun and goes a-hunting!

The Movie Murderer (1970): A man whose hobby is setting fire to aircraft is caught on film, and recognized by an insurance detective. While the arsonist hunts the film negatives, the sleuth hunts him.

Panic on the 5:22 (1974): Juvenile delinquents hound commuters in a railroad bar car.

Writers of note who have worked for television:

Rod Sterling: the bulk of his output was for TV, original dramas and episodes of *The Twilight Zone*
Sidney Sheldon: now one of the world's top-selling novelists, he used to write for *I Dream of Jeannie* (and was an Emmy winner for same)
Mel Brooks: the producer-director-writer-actor was once a staff writer for Sid Caesar
Paddy Chayefsky: lauded for *Network, The Hospital, Altered States*, and others, but his best work remains his teleplays like *Marty*
Kurt Vonnegut, Jr.: prior to adapting his own works, or seeing his novels filmed, he wrote half-hour dramas like *Auf Wiedersehen* for the *General Electric Theatre* and others
Neil Simon: like Mel Brooks, he contributed his considerable wit to Sid Caesar
Gore Vidal: before moving on to novels and films like *Caligula*, Vidal wrote *Visit to a Small Planet* for the home tube
Arthur Hailey: like Sheldon, a top-flight commercial novelist, he penned hour-long dramas for live TV in the 1950s

. . . and a few actors who have written for their own series:

Robert Culp (*I Spy*; *The Greatest American Hero*)
Chevy Chase (*Saturday Night Live*)
Alan Alda (*M*A*S*H*)

Wordsmiths (continued)

Steve Allen (*Meeting of Minds*)
Dick Van Dyke (*Van Dyke and Company*)
Patrick McGoohan (*The Prisoner*)
McLean Stevenson (*M*A*S*H*)

The year 1946 was the first "official" season as far as TV historians are concerned. It had a regular schedule, and while the shows were rather unspectacular, this is the seed for which our current fare grew:

Face to Face
Geographically Speaking
Esso Newsreel
Voice of Firestone
Gillette Cavalcade of Sports
Play the Game
Television Screen Magazine
Serving Through Science
Let's Rhumba
Cash and Carry
Faraway Hill
Hour Glass
I Love to Eat
The World in Your Home

The last, ironically, was not only a show but a forecast of what the new medium was soon to become!

ABOUT THE AUTHOR

JEFF ROVIN, a workaholic and confirmed movie fan, now in his mid-twenties, was born in Brooklyn and raised on Long Island. After two years in college he dropped out to enter the field of publishing, working as a comic-book editor and even writing a romance column. His first book, *A Pictorial History of Science Fiction Films,* was followed by twelve others, including *The UFO Movie Quiz Book, The Superhero Movie & TV Quiz Book, Count Dracula's Vampire Quiz Book,* the last three in Signet paperback; *The Films of Charlton Heston, The Great Television Series,* and others. He is a frequent guest lecturer, speaking on science fiction, films, and movie effects, writes a column for *Analog* magazine, and articles for *Ladies Home Journal.*